Single Best Answer MCQs in

ANAESTHESIA

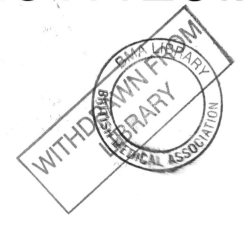

Volume II Basic Sciences

Cyprian Mendonca, Mahesh Chaudhari, Arumugam Pitchiah

tfm Publishing Limited, Castle Hill Barns, Harley, Nr Shrewsbury, SY5 6LX, UK. Tel: +44 (0)1952 510061; Fax: +44 (0)1952 510192 E-mail: nikki@tfmpublishing.com; Web site: www.tfmpublishing.com

Design & Typesetting: Nikki Bramhill BSc Hons Dip Law
First Edition: © September 2011
Background cover image © Comstock Inc., www.comstock.com

ISBN: 978 1 903378 83 0

Printed by Gutenberg Press Ltd., Gudja Road, Tarxien, PLA 19, Malta. Tel: +356 21897037; Fax: +356 21800069.

ii

Contents

		Page
Preface		iv
Acknowledgements		vi
Abbreviations		viii
Set 1	Questions	1
Set 1	Answers	13
Set 2	Questions	33
Set 2	Answers	45
Set 3	Questions	69
Set 3	Answers	81
Set 4	Questions	103
Set 4	Answers	113
Set 5	Questions	135
Set 5	Answers	147
Set 6	Questions	169
Set 6	Answers	181

Preface

Single best answer type multiple choice questions have been introduced into anaesthetic postgraduate examinations as a way of assessing the trainee's ability to apply knowledge to clinical practice. Although this is more relevant for topics in clinical anesthesia, recently this method of assessment has been extended to topics in basic sciences.

This book consists of six sets of single best answer practice papers. Each set comprises 30 multiple choice questions drawn from physiology, pharmacology, clinical measurement, equipment and physics relevant to anaesthetic examinations. Each question consists of a stem describing a clinical scenario or problem followed by five possible answer options. One of them is the best response for the given question. Each question and answer is accompanied by supporting notes obtained from peer-reviewed journal articles and basic science textbooks. Alongside the previously published book *Single Best Answer MCQs in Anaesthesia* (Volume I – Clinical Anaesthesia, ISBN 978-1-903378-75-5), this book supplements the essential study material for postgraduate anaesthetic examinations.

The main objective of this book is to provide trainees with a series of single best answer type questions that will prepare them for this format of postgraduate examinations. Much emphasis has been placed on the understanding and application of basic science knowledge with regards to clinical practice.

We hope that a thorough revision of this book will enable trainees to improve their understanding and core knowledge of basic sciences relevant to anaesthesia. We believe this book will not only be an invaluable educational resource for those who are preparing for postgraduate examinations, but will also be of benefit to any practising anaesthetist.

Cyprian Mendonca MD, FRCA
Consultant Anaesthetist
University Hospitals Coventry and Warwickshire
Coventry, UK

Mahesh Chaudhari MD, FRCA, FFPMRCA
Consultant Anaesthetist
Worcestershire Royal Hospital
Worcester, UK

Arumugam Pitchiah MD, FRCA
Specialty Registrar
Welsh School of Anaesthesia
Wales, UK

v

Acknowledgements

We are grateful to Dr Jennie Kerr and Dr Clare Ingram, both Specialty Registrars, Warwickshire School of Anaesthesia, who critically reviewed the entire manuscript and made suggestions for improvement of the book.

We gratefully acknowledge the help received from Nikki Bramhill, Director, tfm publishing, in reviewing the manuscript.

We extend our thanks to the following who contributed questions to this book:

Dr S Pradeep Angadi
Specialty Registrar, East Midlands (South) School of Anaesthesia

Dr Shefali Chaudhari
Specialty Registrar, Warwickshire School of Anaesthesia

Dr Smita Gohil
Specialty Registrar, Warwickshire School of Anaesthesia

Dr Kate Henderson
Specialty Registrar, Birmingham School of Anaesthesia

Dr Carl Hillermann
Consultant Anaesthetist, University Hospital, Coventry

Dr Payal Kajekar
Specialty Registrar, Warwickshire School of Anaesthesia

Dr Raja Lakshmanan
Consultant Anaesthetist, Queen Elizabeth Hospital, Birmingham

Dr Deepak Malik
Specialty Registrar, East Midlands (South) School of Anaesthesia

Dr Priya Nair
Specialty Registrar, Warwickshire School of Anaesthesia

Dr Shanmugam Paramasivan
Specialty Registrar, Warwickshire School of Anaesthesia

Dr Ganesh K Ramalingam
Specialty Registrar, Warwickshire School of Anaesthesia

Dr Rathinavel Shanmugam
Specialty Registrar, Warwickshire School of Anaesthesia

Dr Rebecca Smith
Specialty Registrar, St. George's School of Anaesthesia

Abbreviations

AAGBI	Association of Anaesthetists of Great Britain and Ireland
ACE	Angiotensin-converting enzyme
ACTH	Adrenocorticotrophic hormone
ADH	Anti-diuretic hormone
ALA	δ-aminolevulinic acid
AOP	Apnoea of prematurity
APTT	Activated partial thromboplastin time
ARDS	Acute respiratory distress syndrome
ASA	American Society of Anesthesiologists
AST	Aspartate transaminase
BD	Twice a day
BP	Blood pressure
cAMP	Cyclic adenosine monophosphate
CBF	Cerebral blood flow
CI	Cardiac index
CK	Creatine kinase
Cl	Chloride
CMR	Cerebral metabolic rate
CNS	Central nervous system
CO	Carbon monoxide
CO	Cardiac output
COAD	Chronic obstructive airway disease
COPD	Chronic obstructive pulmonary disease
CPAP	Continuous positive airway pressure
CPP	Cerebral perfusion pressure
CPR	Cardiopulmonary resuscitation
CSF	Cerebrospinal fluid
CSWS	Cerebral salt wasting syndrome
CT	Computed tomography
CVP	Central venous pressure

DPG	2,3-diphosphoglycerate
EBV	Estimated blood volume
ECF	Extracellular fluid
ECG	Electrocardiogram
EDV	End-diastolic volume
EEG	Electro-encephalography
EF	Ejection fraction
ESR	Erythrocyte sedimentation rate
ESV	End-systolic volume
$EtCO_2$	End-tidal CO_2
FEUA	Fractional excretion of uric acid
FEV	Forced expiratory volume
FFA	Free fatty acids
FGF	Fresh gas flow
FRC	Functional residual capacity
FVC	Forced vital capacity
GA	General anaesthesia
GTN	Glyceryl trinitrate
H	Hydrogen
Hb	Haemoglobin
HBO	Hyperbaric oxygen
HCO_3	Bicarbonate
HME	Heat-moisture exchange
HPV	Hypoxic pulmonary vasoconstriction
IABP	Intra-aortic balloon pump
IBW	Ideal body weight
ICF	Intracellular fluid
ICP	Intracranial pressure
ICU	Intensive care unit
IV	Intravenous
K	Potassium
LA	Local anaesthesia
LDH	Lactic dehydrogenase
LMA	Laryngeal mask airway
LMWH	Low-molecular-weight heparin
MABL	Maximum allowable blood loss
MAC	Minimum alveolar concentration
MAOI	Monoamine oxidase inhibitor
MAP	Mean arterial pressure
MRA	Magnetic resonance angiography

MRI	Magnetic resonance imaging
MST	Morphine sulphate
Na	Sodium
NMB	Neuromuscular block
NSAID	Non-steroidal anti-inflammatory drug
OD	Once a day
PAP	Pulmonary artery pressure
PAWP	Pulmonary artery wedge pressure
PCT	Proximal convoluted tubule
PCV	Packed cell volume
PDE	Phosphodiesterase
PDPH	Postdural puncture headache
PEEP	Positive end expiratory pressure
PMR	Polymyalgia rheumatica
PONV	Postoperative nausea and vomiting
PT	Prothrombin time
PTH	Parathyroid hormone
PVR	Pulmonary vascular resistance
PVRI	Pulmonary vascular resistance index
RBC	Red blood cell
RV	Residual volume
SIADH	Syndrome of inappropriate anti-diuretic hormone secretion
SLN	Superior laryngeal nerve
STP	Standard temperature and pressure
SVP	Saturated vapour pressure
SVR	Systemic vascular resistance
SVRI	Systemic vascular resistance index
TBW	Total body water
TCA	Tricyclic antidepressant
TCI	Target controlled infusion
TDS	Three times a day
TEF	Tracheo-oesophageal fistulae
TOE	Transoesophageal echocardiogram
TOF	Train of four
TPN	Total parenteral nutrition
TRH	Thyrotropin releasing hormone
TSH	Thyroid stimulating hormone
VAE	Venous air embolism
VIE	Vacuum-insulated evaporator
VSD	Ventricular septal defect

Set 1 questions

1 Which of the following is the most effective process to maintain an energy supply to muscles during physical exertion in trained athletes (as compared to untrained individuals)?

a. Protein catabolism.
b. Effective utilisation of free fatty acids.
c. More glycogen utilisation.
d. More lactate production.
e. Gluconeogenesis by deamination.

2 A 47-year-old female is due to undergo a hysterectomy. Her pre-operative ECG shows progressive lengthening of the PR interval until a ventricular beat is dropped. Which of the following conduction abnormalities is she most likely to have?

a. First degree heart block.
b. Mobitz type 1 heart block.
c. Mobitz type 2 heart block.
d. Left bundle branch block.
e. Right bundle branch block.

3 Hypoxic pulmonary vasoconstriction (HPV) in the lungs is a compensatory mechanism to improve ventilation perfusion

matching. In which of the following would a decrease most likely trigger HPV?

a.   Partial pressure of oxygen in the pulmonary artery.
b.   Partial pressure of oxygen in the pulmonary veins.
c.   Partial pressure of oxygen in the alveoli.
d.   Oxygen saturation of haemoglobin in the pulmonary artery.
e.   Oxygen saturation of haemoglobin in the pulmonary veins.

4   You perform an uncomplicated lumbar epidural for labour analgesia on a 27-year-old lady of 36 weeks' gestation with twins. Immediately after the test dose of 15ml 0.25% bupivacaine she lies supine and her BP is 70/40. The most likely cause for hypotension in this patient is:

a.   Concealed ante-partum haemorrhage.
b.   Intrathecal injection of local anaesthetic.
c.   Dehydration.
d.   Aorto-caval compression.
e.   Anaphylaxis.

5   A 35-year-old patient with a BMI of 35 aspirates gastric contents on induction of anaesthesia. One week later on the ICU, a diagnosis of acute respiratory distress syndrome is made. Which of the following mechanisms is most likely to contribute to the associated pulmonary oedema?

a.   Increased pulmonary capillary permeability.
b.   Raised pulmonary capillary hydrostatic pressure due to fluid overload.
c.   Reduced lymphatic drainage.
d.   Reduced alveolar interstitial pressure.
e.   Decreased oncotic pressure in the pulmonary capillary.

6   A 29-year-old woman on lithium for bipolar disease was brought to the emergency department where she was found to be unresponsive. She has a history of convulsions and her ECG shows conduction defects with ST changes. Plasma lithium levels were found to be 7.5mmol/L. In addition to supportive treatment, specific management would be:

a.   Haemodialysis.
b.   Administration of magnesium.
c.   Forced alkaline diuresis.
d.   Acetazolamide administration.
e.   Diazepam infusion.

7   A 66-year-old male with hypertension and ischemic heart disease is scheduled for an open cholecystectomy. The best technique among the following to suppress the pressor response to laryngoscopy and intubation would be:

a.   Intravenous esmolol.
b.   Morphine 0.4mg/kg prior to intubation.
c.   Isoflurane.
d.   Intravenous phentolamine.
e.   GTN spray prior to induction.

8   A 53-year-old woman suffering from chronic back pain presents for excision of a small lipoma on the forearm under general anaesthesia. Her regular medication includes 100mg of morphine sulphate continuous twice daily. In the postoperative period the optimal dose of oral morphine to be prescribed would be:

a.   20mg every 4 hours with extra doses of 20mg for breakthrough pain.
b.   30mg every 4 hours with extra doses of 30mg for breakthrough pain.
c.   20mg every 6 hours with extra doses of 20mg for breakthrough pain.
d.   30mg every 8 hours with extra doses of 30mg for breakthrough pain.
e.   30mg every 2 hours with extra doses of 30mg for breakthrough pain.

3

9 A 9-year-old boy weighing 40kg is undergoing an appendicectomy. He became severely hypotensive 5 minutes after the administration of an antibiotic. He developed a rash all over his body. His blood pressure is 65/45mmHg, his heart rate is 140 per minute and he has weak central pulses. The most appropriate dose and route of administering adrenaline is:

a.   0.1ml/kg of 1:10 000 adrenaline IV.
b.   0.1ml/kg of 1:100 000 adrenaline IV.
c.   0.1ml/kg of 1:1000 adrenaline IV.
d.   0.1ml/kg of 1:10 000 adrenaline IM.
e.   0.1ml/kg of 1: 20 000 adrenaline IM.

10 A 47-year-old woman is scheduled for an elective total abdominal hysterectomy. She consents for a lumbar epidural for postoperative analgesia. In the anaesthetic room, at 10am, it is noted from her prescription chart that she has had a prophylactic dose of enoxaparin the previous evening at 22:00 hours. The best management option is:

a.   To avoid the epidural and choose an alternative method of postoperative analgesia.
b.   To continue with the scheduled plan of epidural analgesia.
c.   To postpone surgery to another day.
d.   To estimate anti-Xa levels prior to insertion.
e.   To review PT and APTT prior to insertion.

11 A patient is receiving oxygen at a rate of 10L/minute, from a size E cylinder (volume 5L). The pressure in the cylinder is 100 bar. How long can oxygen be delivered from this cylinder?

a.   30 minutes.
b.   40 minutes.
c.   45 minutes.
d.   50 minutes.
e.   60 minutes.

12 You are starting the first case on a Sunday morning in the emergency theatre. After induction of general anaesthesia, despite adequate mask ventilation using 6L/minute of oxygen flow, the oxygen saturation begins to fall. The oxygen analyser at the common gas outlet (fuel cell) and at the mask end of the breathing system (paramagnetic analyser) reads inspired oxygen concentration as 21%. Despite turning the oxygen cylinder on (pressure reads 90 bar), the oxygen saturation continues to fall. The single most important next step in the management is:

a. Immediate tracheal intubation.
b. Ventilate using a resuscitation bag and auxiliary oxygen source from the same anaesthetic machine.
c. Change the pulse oximeter probe.
d. Disconnect the oxygen pipeline.
e. Change the oxygen cylinder on the machine.

13 A 60-year-old male patient is ventilated using volume-controlled ventilation. The normal waveform of $EtCO_2$ gradually (over 15 minutes) changes to the following trace (Figure 1). Which of the following situations best describes the change in the $EtCO_2$ waveform?

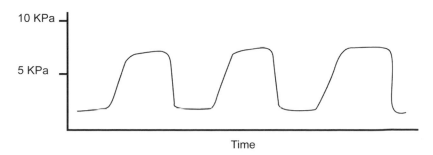

Figure 1. Volume-controlled ventilation $EtCO_2$ waveform.

a. Spontaneous breathing.
b. Hypoventilation.
c. Malfunction of inspiratory valve.
d. Malfunction of expiratory valve.
e. Exhaustion of CO_2 absorber.

14 The figure below is an arterial trace from a 70-year-old patient with chronic obstructive airway disease, in the intensive care unit. This trace indicates:

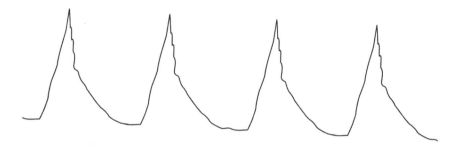

Figure 2. Arterial trace.

a. Presence of blood clot in the cannula.
b. An under-damped trace.
c. Compliant tubing.
d. Atrial fibrillation.
e. Kinking of the cannula.

15 You are planning to perform a gas induction with sevoflurane (molecular weight = 200 and density = 1.5). The vaporiser dial is set at 6%, with a fresh gas flow of 5L/minute using a Mapleson A breathing system. How much liquid sevoflurane is required for the first 5 minutes?

a. 3ml.
b. 5ml.
c. 7ml.
d. 9ml.
e. 11ml.

16 A 27-year-old man is keen to climb up to the summit of Mount Everest without using additional oxygen. Which of the following is the most significant physiological adaptation for his successful acclimatization?

a. Increase in 2,3-DPG in red blood cells.
b. Improved ventilation perfusion matching.
c. Hyperventilation.
d. Polycythaemia.
e. Improved ability of the body to generate energy from anaerobic metabolism.

17 A female patient with a BMI of 49 is scheduled to undergo gastric banding surgery. A change in which of the following parameters confers the greatest advantage when pre-oxygenating her in the sitting (rather than supine) position?

a. Vital capacity.
b. Ventilation/perfusion matching.
c. Tidal volume.
d. Closing capacity.
e. Functional residual capacity.

18 A 39-year-old lady was admitted to intensive care from a medical ward where she was treated for pneumonia and diabetes mellitus. She is intubated and ventilated. Two hours following intensive treatment the following parameters were observed (Table 1).

Table 1. Vital parameters.	
HR	126/minute
BP	80/44 (55)mmHg,
CVP	+5mmHg
Body surface area	2m^2
Cardiac output	8L/min
Stroke volume	80ml
PA pressure	25/7(13)mmHg
PAWP	6mmHg
SvO$_2$	65%
CaO$_2$	15ml.dl-1

Her systemic vascular resistance would be:

a. 400dynes.s.cm^{-5}.
b. 500dynes.s.cm^{-5}.
c. 550dynes.s.cm^{-5}.
d. 600dynes.s.cm^{-5}.
e. 650dynes.s.cm^{-5}.

19 A 70-year-old male patient with severe chronic obstructive airway disease has been intubated and ventilated in the intensive care unit. Before intubation and ventilation his oxygen saturation was 90%; it is now 100%. His PaO$_2$ has increased from 8kPa to 20kPa. His haemoglobin is 15g/dL and pH is 7.32. His oxygen content in the blood is:

a. Increased by 15ml/100ml.
b. Increased by 12ml/100ml.
c. Increased by 9ml/100ml.
d. Increased by 6ml/100ml.
e. Increased by 3ml/100ml.

20 A 70-year-old man is scheduled for a knee arthroplasty. Prior to induction of general anaesthesia a femoral nerve block is performed using a nerve stimulator. Soon after injection of 20ml of 0.5% bupivacaine, he became unresponsive. He is unconscious and has no palpable carotid pulse. CPR is commenced. Which one of the following best describes the specific treatment in this scenario?

a. 1ml/kg of 10% lipid emulsion over 1 minute.
b. 1.5ml/kg of 20% lipid emulsion over 1 minute.
c. 1.5ml/kg of 20% lipid emulsion over 5 minutes.
d. 1ml/kg of 10% lipid emulsion over 1 minute.
e. 1.5ml/kg of 10% lipid emulsion over 2 minutes.

21 In a 40-year-old male (total body water of this patient is 60L) after oral administration and absorption, drug A is distributed only in extracellular fluid. If the terminal half-life of the drug is 500 minutes, which one of the following most closely represents the clearance value (ml/minute) for this drug?

a. 14.
b. 28.
c. 20.
d. 34.
e. 40.

22 A 38-year-old woman with a body mass index of 48 is to undergo an elective laparotomy for gynaecological surgery. The induction dose of propofol is best calculated based on:

a. Actual body weight.
b. Ideal body weight.
c. Lean body mass.
d. Body mass index.
e. Ideal body weight + 20% total body weight.

23 A 11-year-old obese girl has undergone a tonsillectomy. Later that evening she is found pale and hypotensive. She is diagnosed with post-tonsillectomy bleeding. She is very anxious. The preferred method of induction would be:

a. Inhalational induction with sevoflurane with a head-down tilt.
b. Rapid sequence induction with thiopentone and suxamethonium.
c. Rapid sequence induction with thiopentone and rocuronium.
d. Rapid sequence induction with propofol and rocuronium.
e. Inhalational induction with desflurane with a head-down tilt.

24 A 35-year-old woman is brought to the emergency department following a suspected amitriptyline overdose. She has a GCS of 6 and her blood pressure is 90/46mmHg. A 12-lead ECG is recorded; it is highly likely to show:

a. Atrial fibrillation.
b. Sinus bradycardia with a prolonged QRS complex.
c. Sinus tachycardia with a prolonged QRS complex.
d. Complete heart block.
e. Ventricular tachycardia.

25 A 40-year-old ASA 1 male patient with a body mass index of 28 is undergoing a complex orthopaedic procedure on the left forearm lasting for 8 hours. The most appropriate reason for choosing

invasive arterial blood pressure monitoring over automated non-invasive blood pressure measurement in this patient is:

a. Automated non-invasive blood pressure monitoring would be inaccurate in this patient.
b. Automated blood pressure monitoring is likely to result in ulnar nerve injury.
c. Monitoring invasive blood pressure ensures adequate perfusion pressure.
d. Hypotension can be detected early using invasive blood pressure monitoring.
e. Automated non-invasive blood pressure monitoring for 8 hours can result in distal oedema of the limb.

26 You encountered a difficult laryngoscopy in a patient scheduled for an emergency laparotomy. The laryngoscopic view was grade 3. You managed to intubate the trachea by railroading the tracheal tube over a gum elastic bougie. Which of the following is the most reliable method of confirming the correct placement of the tracheal tube?

a. Feeling clicks whilst advancing the bougie.
b. Distal hold up of bougie.
c. Presence of CO_2 in the initial few breaths.
d. Presence of bilateral chest movement.
e. Endoscopic confirmation using a fibreoptic scope.

27 A 65-year-old male patient presents with severe shortness of breath due to extrinsic compression of the mid-trachea. Which of the following statements best describes the reason for administering heliox in this patient?

a. It decreases the density of the gas mixture.
b. It decreases the viscosity of the gas mixture.
c. It decreases the Reynold's number.
d. It converts turbulent flow into laminar flow.
e. It decreases the friction coefficient of the gas mixture.

28 You discover that an anaesthetic machine with a sodalime absorber and a desflurane vaporiser has not been used for the last 48 hours. However, the fresh gas flow was left running at 2L/minute for the last 48 hours. Which of the following is the most appropriate action before using this machine to administer anaesthesia to the first patient on the list?

a. Use a different anaesthetic machine.
b. Change the sodalime absorber and use the same anaesthetic machine.
c. Continuously flush the anaesthetic machine for 1 hour and then use the machine.
d. Use high fresh gas flow for the first hour.
e. Change the vaporiser to isoflurane.

29 A 4-year-old child weighing 16kg is scheduled for an inguinal herniotomy. You are planning to maintain the airway using a laryngeal mask airway (LMA). Which of the following is the most suitably sized LMA for this child?

a. Size 1½.
b. Size 2.
c. Size 2½.
d. Size 3.
e. Size 3½.

30 At the end of an elective right hemicolectomy, it is noticed that the heat-moisture exchange (HME) filter was not used during the entire procedure. Four days later the patient develops a lower respiratory tract infection. Which of the following mechanisms initiates the cascade of events leading to respiratory tract infection in this patient?

a. Evaporation of water from mucus lining the epithelium of the trachea.
b. Loss of the mucociliary elevator mechanism.
c. The change in the isothermic saturation boundary within the airways.
d. Viscous secretions gradually occluding the tracheal tube.
e. Hypothermia resulting from the use of dry and cool inspired gas.

Set 1 answers

1 Answer: B. Effective utilisation of free fatty acids.

Trained athletes are able to increase the oxygen consumption of their muscles to a greater degree than untrained individuals and are able to utilise free fatty acids more effectively. Therefore, they are capable of greater exertion without depleting their glycogen store and increasing their lactate production. Protein catabolism or deamination occurs during starvation and is not the usual process by which energy is derived during exercise. Glycogenolysis occurs during exertion as a routine both in trained and untrained individuals.

Further reading
1. Bastiaans JJ, van Diemen AB, Veneberg T, Jeukendrup AE. The effects of replacing a portion of endurance training by explosive strength training on performance in trained cyclists. *European Journal of Applied Physiology* 2001; 86: 79-84.

2 Answer: B. Mobitz type 1 heart block.

Conduction blocks in the heart can be classified as incomplete, when conduction between the atria and ventricles is slowed but not completely interrupted, and complete block.

In first degree heart block, all the atrial impulses reach the ventricles but the PR interval is abnormally long. In second degree heart block, not all atrial impulses are conducted to the ventricles. In Mobitz type 1 block, the PR interval lengthens progressively until a ventricular beat is dropped, also called the Wenckebach phenomenon. In Mobitz type 2 block, not all atrial impulses are conducted to the ventricles. There may be a ventricular beat following only every second or third atrial beat (2:1 or 3:1 block).

Further reading
1. Silverman ME, Upshaw CB Jr, Lange HW. Woldemar Mobitz and His 1924 classification of second-degree atrioventricular block. *Circulation* 2004; 110: 1162-7.

3   Answer: C. Partial pressure of oxygen in the alveoli.

Hypoxic pulmonary vasoconstriction (HPV) helps to divert blood flow from non-ventilated areas to ventilated areas of the lungs, and therefore improves ventilation perfusion matching. It is the partial pressure of oxygen in the alveoli which has most effect on adjacent blood vessels leading to vasoconstriction. HPV mainly occurs in small pre-capillary arterioles; the overall increase in pulmonary vascular resistance remains less than 20%.

Further reading
1. Naeije R, Brimioulle S. Physiology in medicine: importance of hypoxic pulmonary vasoconstriction in maintaining arterial oxygenation during acute respiratory failure. *Crit Care* 2001; 5: 67-71.

4   Answer: D. Aorto-caval compression.

Significant hypotension in the supine position in a pregnant female is most likely to be due to aorto-caval compression. Intrathecal injection of 15ml of 0.25% bupivacaine in a female of 36 weeks' gestation is likely to cause unrecordable blood pressure with severe bradycardia or cardiac arrest. Concealed haemorrhage or dehydration will not lead to a sudden drop in blood pressure and anaphylaxis will be associated with other features such as tachycardia, bronchospasm and rash.

Further reading
1. Dresner M, Bamber JH. Aortocaval compression in pregnancy: the effect of changing the degree and direction of lateral tilt on maternal cardiac output. *Anaesthesia and Analgesia* 2003; 97: 256-8.

5   Answer: A. Increased pulmonary capillary permeability.

Acute respiratory distress syndrome (ARDS) is a known complication following aspiration. Inflammatory changes in the lungs lead to increased alveolar capillary permeability and reduced surfactant production causing pulmonary oedema. Alveolar interstitial pressure may rise in ARDS due to the collapse of alveoli.

Further reading
1. Ware L, Matthay M. The acute respiratory distress syndrome. *New England Journal of Medicine* 2000; 342: 1334-49.

6   Answer: A. Haemodialysis.

Haemodialysis is the treatment of choice. This lady probably has an acute on chronic overdose since she is on lithium therapy. Plasma levels should be obtained immediately, at 6 hours and at 12 hours.

Haemodialysis is the definitive treatment when the plasma level of lithium exceeds 7.5mmol/L in an acute overdose or 4.0mmol/L in an acute on chronic overdose. Forced alkaline diuresis is contraindicated. A benzodiazepine infusion can be used only as a measure to control seizures. Acetazolamide and magnesium do not have a role to play in the management.

Further reading
1. Flood S, Bodenham A. Lithium: mimicry, mania and muscle relaxants. *British Journal of Anaesthesia CEACCP* 2010; 10: 77-80.
2. Jephcott G, Kerry RJ. Lithium: an anesthetic risk. *British Journal of Anaesthesia* 1974; 46: 389-90.

7   Answer: A. Intravenous esmolol.

Esmolol is a short-acting cardioselective β1-adrenergic blocker with a rapid onset of action. It is very effective in controlling the pressor response to intubation. Morphine can blunt the cardiovascular response, but not as effectively as esmolol. Adequate depth of anaesthesia using isoflurane is helpful in minimising the cardiovascular response to intubation. GTN infusions have been tried to control the pressor response to intubation, but a sublingual spray is not effective. Phentolamine is an α-adrenoreceptor blocker usually used to treat hypertension associated with activation of α-adrenorecptors such as in pheochromocytoma.

The following techniques can be used to suppress the laryngoscopic response:

◆ Esmolol: 0.5mg/kg over 30 seconds prior to laryngoscopy.
◆ Alfentanil: 20-30µg/kg 1 minute prior to laryngoscopy.
◆ Remifentanil: 0.5µg/kg bolus prior to laryngoscopy.
◆ Additional dose of propofol 0.5mg/kg prior to laryngoscopy.
◆ Lidocaine: 1.5mg/kg prior to laryngoscopy.
◆ Ensuring adequate muscle relaxation by monitoring the response to neuromuscular stimulation.

Further reading
1. Singh H, Vichitvejpaisal P, Gaines GY, White PF. Comparative effects of lidocaine, esmolol and nitroglycerine in modifying the haemodynamic response to laryngoscopy and intubation. *J Clin Anesth* 1995; 7: 5-8.
2. Kovac AL. Controlling the haemodynamic response to laryngoscopy and endotracheal intubation. *J Clin Anesth* 1996; 8: 63-79.

8   Answer: B. 30mg every 4 hours with extra doses of 30mg for breakthrough pain.

This lady is on 100mg twice daily dosage. The baseline morphine requirement over 24 hours is 200mg. This patient should be able to take morphine orally after surgery as this is a minor procedure. The 4-hourly oral morphine dose can be calculated (200/6) = 30mg every 4 hours and the remainder can be administered as 30mg PRN.

A 20mg dose is too small and would not meet her baseline requirements, whilst 6 or 8 hours in between subsequent doses is unnecessary and would not provide good plasma concentrations for analgesia.

If unable to take 30mg orally then she can be prescribed either IV morphine or subcutaneous morphine. The oral to IV morphine conversion would be 3:1 approximately (33% oral bioavailability), while the oral to subcutaneous conversion would be 4:1 approximately. For example, if a patient is taking 120mg/day of oral morphine, he/she would require 40mg/day of intravenous morphine.

Further reading
1. Stannard C, Booth S. Practical guide to opioid therapy - cancer pain. In: *Churchill's pocketbook of pain*, 2nd ed. Philadelphia, USA: Elsevier Churchill Livingstone, 2004; Section 2, Chapter 12: 229-47.

9   Answer: B. 0.1ml/kg of 1:100,000 adrenaline IV.

The clinical features are suggestive of anaphylaxis. According to the AAGBI guideline, children may be given an intravenous dose of adrenaline if they are in a properly monitored area where expertise is available, such as the operating theatre or intensive care unit.

The dose of adrenaline in anaphylaxis in children is 1µg/kg IV (0.1ml/kg of 1:100,000).

The intramuscular route is preferred where there is no venous access or where establishing venous access would cause a delay in drug administration.

Further reading
1. Association of Anaesthetists of Great Britain and Ireland. Suspected anaphylactic reactions associated with anaesthesia. *Anaesthesia* 2009; 64: 199-211.

10   Answer: B. To continue with the scheduled plan of epidural analgesia.

The patient has been given a dose of prophylactic low-molecular-weight heparin the evening before the surgery. A neuraxial blockade can be performed, or an epidural catheter removed 12 hours after administration of low-molecular-weight heparin. Therefore, in this patient, an epidural block can be performed safely at 10:00 hours on the morning of surgery. There is no need to postpone the surgery to a different day.

The estimation of anti-Xa levels, prothrombin time (PT) or activated partial thromboplastin time (APTT) levels would add no useful information to arrive at a decision.

Further reading
1. Conn D, Nicholls B. Anticoagulation and regional anaesthesia - regional anaesthesia. In: *Oxford handbook of anaesthesia*. Almann KG, Wilson IH, Eds. Oxford, UK: Oxford University Press, 2006; Chapter 41: 1058-60.
2. Horlocker TT, *et al*. Regional anaesthesia in the anticoagulated patient. Defining the risks (the second ASRA Consensus Conference on Neuraxial Anaesthesia and Anticoagulation). *Reg Anesth Pain Med* 2003; 28: 172-97.

11   Answer: D. 50 minutes.

A full-size E oxygen cylinder (137 bar pressure) contains 680L of oxygen. In the given cylinder the pressure is reduced to 100 bar indicating that it is partially empty. According to Boyle's law, the volume of oxygen in the cylinder can be estimated by measuring the pressure within the cylinder. At 100 bar pressure, a 5L cylinder contains 500L of oxygen. At a gas flow of 10L/minute, it could deliver oxygen for 50 minutes.

Further reading
1. Davis PD, Kenny GNC. The gas laws. In: *Basic physics and measurement in anaesthesia*, 5th ed. London, UK: Butterworth-Heinemann, 2003: 37-50.

12   Answer: D. Disconnect the oxygen pipeline.

It is very unlikely that both oxygen analysers (fuel cell and paramagnetic analyser) are faulty. Therefore, for some reason 21% oxygen (air) is being delivered to the patient. The most likely reason is the pipelines have been swapped over and the oxygen pipeline is delivering air.

Some anaesthetic machines have a pipeline preference by setting the cylinder pressure regulators to 350kPa (50 psi), in which case even if the cylinder is turned on gases will be delivered from the pipeline. This feature is incorporated to prevent the premature emptying of the cylinder when the reserve cylinder is accidentally left turned on. Hence, disconnecting the pipeline allows the anaesthetic machine to deliver oxygen from the reserve cylinder.

Immediate tracheal intubation is not required, as the patient is being adequately ventilated using a bag and mask. If the pipeline is not disconnected, the auxiliary oxygen source will also deliver 21% oxygen.

Further reading
1. Diba A. The anaesthetic. In: *Ward's anaesthetic equipment*, 5th ed, Davey AJ, Diba A, Eds. Philadelphia, USA: Elsevier Saunders, 2005; Chapter 6: 91-30.
2. Brockwell RC, Andrews JJ. Anaesthesia work station pneumatics. In: *Miller's anesthesia,* volume 1, 7th ed. Miller RD, Ed. Philadelphia, USA: Churchill Livingstone, 2010; Chapter 25: 674-83.

13 Answer: E. Exhaustion of CO_2 absorber.

The capnograph trace shows an elevated inspiratory baseline. In a normal trace the inspiratory baseline should be zero. The most likely causes are malfunction of the expiratory valve and an exhausted sodalime absorber allowing rebreathing of CO_2. Since the waveform is gradually changed, it is unlikely to be due to expiratory valve malfunction. This abnormal waveform is common in clinical practice, when low-flow anaesthesia is used. Monitoring change in the inspiratory baseline is useful in detecting rebreathing of CO_2. Hypoventilation would result in elevation of $EtCO_2$ without changing the inspiratory baseline. Similarly, spontaneous breathing does not affect the inspiratory baseline.

Further reading
1. Bhavani-Shankar K, Mosley H, Kumar AY. Capnometry and anaesthesia, review article. *Canadian Journal of Anaesthesia* 1992; 39: 617-32.

14   Answer: B. An under-damped trace.

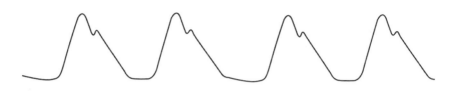

Figure 1. A normal arterial waveform.

The arterial trace presented in the question shows a falsely high systolic pressure and a falsely low diastolic pressure. The mean arterial pressure is unaffected. An under-damped arterial trace is recognised by the presence of an overshoot spike (ringing). Increased resonance can be due to a stiff, non-compliant diaphragm and tubing. The waveform is under-damped.

Over-damping (damping) results in a smoothed out trace without displaying sharp changes, leading to under-reading of systolic pressure and over-reading of diastolic pressure. The loss of pressure in the fluid-filled tubing system, soft compliant tubing, numerous connections and stopcocks, kinking of the cannula, blood clots and air bubbles can result in an over-damped arterial trace.

Further reading
1.   Bedford RF, Shah NK. Blood pressure monitoring. In: *Monitoring in anaesthesia and critical care*, 3rd ed. Blitt CD, Hines RL, Eds. New York, USA: Churchill Livingstone, 1995; 95-130.

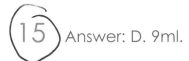 Answer: D. 9ml.

Avogadro's hypothesis states that 1g mole of liquid when vaporised occupies 22.4L at standard temperature and pressure (STP). The molecular weight of sevoflurane is 200g, hence 200g of sevoflurane produces 22.4L of vapour at STP. The density of sevoflurane is 1.5. Therefore (200/1.5 = 133.33), 133ml of liquid sevoflurane produces 22.4L of vapour and 1ml of sevoflurane produces 168ml of vapour at 20°C.

6% at 5L/minute would be 300ml of vapour per minute. For 5 minutes, 1500ml of vapour is required. About 9ml of sevoflurane is required to produce 1500ml (1500/168) of vapour.

Further reading
1. Davis PD, Kenny GNC. The gas laws. In: *Basic physics and measurement in anaesthesia*, 5th ed. London, UK: Butterworth-Heinemann, 2003; Chapter 4: 44-6.

16 Answer: D. Polycythaemia.

The human body can adapt to high altitude through immediate and long-term acclimatization. At high altitudes, in the short term, the lack of oxygen is sensed by the chemoreceptor in the carotid body which causes hyperventilation. However, hyperventilation also causes respiratory alkalosis which inhibits the respiratory centre. In addition, at high altitudes the heart rate increases, the stroke volume slightly decreases and non-essential body functions are suppressed.

Full acclimatization requires days or even weeks. Gradually, the body compensates for the respiratory alkalosis by renal excretion of bicarbonate, allowing adequate respiration to provide oxygen without risking alkalosis. It takes about 4 days at any given altitude and is greatly enhanced by acetazolamide. Eventually, the body has lower lactate production (reduced glucose breakdown decreases the amount of lactate formed), decreased plasma volume, increased haematocrit (polycythaemia), increased red blood cell mass, a higher concentration of capillaries in skeletal muscle tissue, increased myoglobin, increased mitochondria, increased aerobic enzyme concentration, an increase in 2,3-diphosphoglycerate (2,3-DPG), hypoxic pulmonary vasoconstriction, and right ventricular hypertrophy.

In the tissues, the number of mitochondria and cytochome oxidase enzyme levels increase, thereby increasing the capacity for oxidative reactions.

Full hematological adaptation to high altitude is achieved when the increase in red blood cells reaches a plateau and stops. After that period, the subject below extreme altitude (5,500 metres [18,000 ft]) is able to perform his activities as if he were at sea level.

Oxygen content is significantly affected by the haemoglobin content of the blood, thus polycythaemia is the most important factor in adaptation at high altitude.

Further reading
1.   Zubieta-Calleja G, Paulev P-E, Zubieta-Calleja L. Zubieta-Castillo G. Altitude adaptation through hematocrit change. *Journal of Physiology and Pharmacology* 2007; 58 (Suppl 5): 811-8.

17   Answer: E. Functional residual capacity.

Functional residual capacity (FRC) is defined as the volume remaining within the lung at the end of normal expiration. It is made up of expiratory reserve volume and residual volume. The functional residual capacity has several important physiological functions. It acts as a reservoir for oxygen; this allows continued oxygenation of the alveolar blood during apnoea and also maintains constant levels throughout the respiratory cycle. It also improves lung compliance and reduces pulmonary vascular resistance.

Functional residual capacity may be reduced by supine positioning, restrictive lung disease or a distended abdomen, due to pregnancy, obesity or bowel obstruction.

Functional residual capacity may be increased by positive end expiratory pressure (PEEP) or continuous positive airway pressure (CPAP), and obstructive airways disease (bronchospasm).

Further reading

1. Rylander C, Hogman M, *et al*. Functional residual capacity and respiratory mechanics as indicators of aeration and collapse in experimental lung injury. *Anaesthesia & Analgesia* 2004; 98(3): 782-9.

18 Answer: B. 500dynes.s.cm^{-5}.

Systemic vascular resistance (SVR) is calculated by using the following formula:

SVR: (MAP-CVP/CO) x 80; (55-5/8) x 80; = 500dynes.s.cm^{-5}

Haemodynamic calculations are shown in Table 1.

Table 1. Haemodynamic calculations.

Pulmonary vascular resistance (PVR): (PAP-PAWP/CO) x 80
Pulmonary vascular resistance index (PVRI): (PAP-PAWP/CI) x 80
Systemic vascular resistance index (SVRI): (MAP-CVP/CI) x 80
DO_2: CO x CaO_2 x 10
CaO_2: Hb x SaO_2 x 1.34/100
Oxygen extraction ratio: CaO_2-CvO_2 / CaO_2

Further reading

1. Gomesall CD, Oh TE. Haemodynamic monitoring. In: *Oh's intensive care manual*, 5th ed. Bersten AD, Soni N, Oh TE, Eds. Philadelphia, USA: Butterworth-Heinemann, 2005: 831-8.

19   Answer: E. Increased by 3ml/100ml.

Oxygen content of the blood can be calculated as follows:

$$\text{Arterial Oxygen Content (ml/100ml)} = \frac{(Hb \times 1.34 \times SaO_2) + (0.023 \times PaO_2)}{100}$$

Where Hb is the haemoglobin, SaO_2 is the percentage of haemoglobin saturated with oxygen and PaO_2 is the partial pressure of arterial oxygen in kPa.

The oxygen delivery (oxygen flux) to the tissues is calculated by multiplying cardiac output (CO) and arterial oxygen content (CaO_2) of the blood.

Prior to intubation, arterial content (ml/100ml) =
(15 x 1.34 x 0.9) + (0.023 x 8)
= 18.09 + 0.18 = 18.27

After intubation, arterial content (ml/100ml) =
(15 x 1.34 x 1) + (0.023 x 20)
= 20.1 + 0.46= 21.02

The difference is 2.75ml/100ml

Further reading
1.   McLellan SA, Walsh TS. Oxygen delivery and haemoglobin. *British Journal of Anaesthesia CEACCP* 2004; 4: 123-6.

20   Answer: B. 1.5ml/kg of 20% lipid emulsion over 1 minute.

The patient has collapsed after the injection of local anaesthetic, hence it is highly likely to be due to local anaesthetic toxicity. As per the AAGBI guideline, an initial intravenous bolus of 20% intralipid, 1.5ml/kg, should be injected over 1 minute. Intravenous propofol cannot be used as a substitute for intralipid emulsion.

Management of local anaesthetic toxicity

- Stop injecting the LA.
- Call for help.
- Maintain the airway and, if necessary, secure it with a tracheal tube.
- Administer 100% oxygen and ensure adequate ventilation (hyperventilation may help by increasing plasma pH in the presence of metabolic acidosis).
- Establish intravenous access.
- Control seizures with benzodiazepine, thiopental or propofol in small incremental doses.
- Specific treatment involves intravenous infusion of intralipid.

An initial intravenous bolus injection of 20% lipid emulsion, 1.5ml/kg, is administered over 1 minute and an intravenous infusion of 20% lipid emulsion is given at 15ml/kg/hour.

A maximum of two repeat boluses (same dose) is given if:

- Cardiovascular stability has not been restored, or
- An adequate circulation deteriorates.

Five minutes should be left between boluses; a maximum of three boluses can be given (including the initial bolus).

The infusion is continued at the same rate, but the rate is doubled to 30ml/kg/hour at any time after 5 minutes, if:

- Cardiovascular stability has not been restored, or
- An adequate circulation deteriorates.

The infusion is continued until the patient is stable and an adequate circulation is restored.

Further reading
1. Association of Anaesthetists of Great Britain and Ireland. Management of severe local anaesthetic toxicity 2. 2010. http://aagbi.org/publications/guidelines/docs/la_toxicity_2010.pdf.

21 Answer: B. 28.

The relationship between the terminal half-life (t ½), volume of distribution (VD) and the clearance (CL) of a drug is explained by the following equation:

$$t\ \tfrac{1}{2} = k \times VD/CL, \text{ where k is a constant (0.693).}$$

The volume of distribution of this drug is equal to the total amount of extracellular fluid (ECF). The ECF is 1/3 of total body water (1/3 of 60,000ml = 20,000ml).

$$CL \times t\ \tfrac{1}{2} = k \times VD = 0.693 \times 20,000 = \sim 14,000$$
$$CL = 14,000/\ t\ \tfrac{1}{2}\ (500)$$
$$CL = 28$$

The volume of distribution is defined as the apparent volume available in the body for the distribution of the drug.

The clearance is defined as the volume of blood or plasma from which a drug would need to be completely removed in unit time in order to account for its elimination from the body.

The terminal half-life is defined as the time required for the plasma concentration to decrease by 50% during the terminal phase of decline.

Further reading
1. Calvey TN, Williams NE. Pharmacokinetics. In: *Principles and practice of pharmacology for anaesthetists*, 4th ed. Oxford, UK: Blackwell Science, 2001; Chapter 2: 22-3.

22 Answer: B. Ideal body weight.

This patient is morbidly obese with a body mass index of 48. Pathophysiological changes in obesity will affect drug distribution and elimination. In morbidly obese patients the induction dose of propofol can be calculated on ideal body weight (IBW). Though propofol is highly lipophilic, it does not accumulate in obese patients, making it suitable for target controlled infusion (TCI) and the dose of propofol for maintenance could be calculated on the same basis as in lean subjects. For maintenance infusions either the total body weight or IBW (0.4 x excess weight) can be used.

IBW is estimated using the formula:

$$IBW \text{ (in kg)} = \text{height (cm)} - X$$
where X is 100 for adult males and 105 for adult females.

Further reading
1. De Baerdemaker LE, Mortier EP, *et al*. Pharmacokinetics in obese patients. *British Journal of Anaesthesia CEACCP* 2004; 4: 152-5.
2. Ogunnaike BO, Jones SB, *et al*. Anesthetic considerations for bariatric surgery. *Anesthesia & Analgesia* 2002; 95: 1793-805.

23 Answer: B. Rapid sequence induction with thiopentone and suxamethonium.

This girl should be considered to have a full stomach, as she could have been swallowing blood. Rapid sequence induction with thiopentone and suxamethonium is generally the preferred method of induction as it enables airway protection, but laryngoscopy may be difficult due to blood and oedema. Propofol may cause significant hypotension in the presence of relative hypovolaemia from bleeding. Although rocuronium may be used for rapid sequence induction, the onset time is greater than suxamethonium, and the return of muscle function is much longer. Inhalational induction in the left lateral or head-down position can also be used; however, it may be complicated with coughing and airway obstruction which may further increase the risk of regurgitation and aspiration.

Further reading
1. Roberts F. Tonsillectomy/adenoidectomy: child - ear, nose and throat surgery. In: *Oxford handbook of anaesthesia*. Oxford, UK; Oxford University Press, 2006; Chapter 25: 612-3.

24 Answer: C. Sinus tachycardia with a prolonged QRS complex.

There are many studies and case reports of ECG patterns seen in tricyclic antidepressant (TCA) overdose. These changes include a prolonged QRS complex, a prolonged QTc interval and right axis deviation. The presence of any ECG changes suggests significant TCA overdose, which may lead to cardiovascular or neurological sequelae. The most common abnormality, however, is sinus tachycardia with a prolonged QRS complex. Sinus bradycardia or varying degrees of heart block may also be found especially in overt metabolic acidosis but are not as common as sinus tachycardia with QRS prolongation.

Further reading
1. Harrigan RA, Brady WJ. ECG abnormalities in tricyclic antidepressant ingestion. *American Journal of Emergency Medicine* 1999; 17: 387-93.

25 Answer: E. Automated non-invasive blood pressure monitoring for 8 hours can result in distal oedema of the limb.

Automated non-invasive blood pressure measurement using a correctly sized cuff is as accurate as invasive measurement. Also, correct positioning with the lower border above the elbow joint prevents any ulnar nerve injury. Delivering adequate perfusion to any organ can be monitored by non-invasive blood pressure measurement. Hypotension can be detected early with the use of shorter cycling times. However, such frequent recordings over a prolonged time predisposes to distal oedema of the limb.

Further reading
1. Hutton P. Monitoring and safety. In: *Fundamental principles and practice of anaesthesia*, 1st ed. Hutton P, Cooper G, James FM, Butterworth J, Eds. London, UK: Martin Dunitz Ltd, 2002; Chapter 12: 164-5.

26 Answer: E. Endoscopic confirmation using a fibreoptic scope.

The methods used for confirming the correct placement of the tracheal tube include repeating direct laryngoscopy, end-tidal CO_2 detection, an oesophageal detector device, and the lung sliding sign using ultrasound and transthoracic impedance. No single technique used for the confirmation of endotracheal tube placement has been proven to be 100% accurate. Whilst visualization of the endotracheal tube passing through the vocal cords represents the primary method for assessing initial endotracheal tube placement, objective confirmation of proper placement is necessary.

End-tidal CO_2 detection has a high sensitivity and specificity but is of no use in patients with circulatory arrest or poor pulmonary circulation. In these patients, delivery of CO_2 to the lungs may be insufficient to produce a reliable confirmation of tube placement.

Bilateral chest movement may indicate bilateral ventilation of the lungs. It is a more subjective sign as compared to endoscopic confirmation. The presence of bilateral chest movement on inspection should be confirmed by another sign such as auscultation or the presence of end-tidal CO_2.

Oesophageal detector devices have some utility as a technique for endotracheal tube position assessment. The presence of a large amount of air in the oesophagus and stomach can result in false positive results. Ultrasound imaging and transthoracic impedance methods offer potential as techniques that may prove to be helpful as adjuncts to detect and monitor the proper location of endotracheal tubes.

Although feeling the clicks and distal hold up are indicators of correct placement of the bougie in the trachea, this does not guarantee the subsequent railroading and correct placement of the tracheal tube.

Endoscopy using a fibreoptic scope not only confirms tracheal intubation, but also excludes endobronchial intubation.

Further reading

1. Sanehi O, Calder I. Capnography and the differentiation between tracheal and oesophageal intubation. *Anaesthesia* 1999; 54: 604-5.

29

27 Answer: A. It decreases the density of the gas mixture.

Gas flow through an obstruction is turbulent which is dependent on the density of the gas. By reducing the density, turbulent flow may become laminar in character and therefore total flow through an orifice can be increased. Substituting nitrogen in the breathing mixture of gases with helium will decrease the density of the gas mixture.

Further reading
1. Ho AMH, Dion PW, Karmakar MK, *et al.* Use of heliox in critical upper airway obstruction. Physiologic and physical considerations in choosing the optimum helium: oxygen mixture. *Resuscitation* 2002; 52: 297-300.

28 Answer: B. Change the sodalime absorber and use the same anaesthetic machine.

Carbon monoxide (CO) can be formed when volatile anaesthetic agents such as desflurane are used with anaesthetic breathing systems containing CO_2 absorbents. The CO production is inversely proportional to the water content of the absorber. It is more of a problem with baralyme than sodalime. The CO production occurs more commonly with desflurane as compared to other volatile agents (desflurane > enflurane > isoflurane and is trivial with halothane and sevoflurane). Severe CO poisoning during desflurane anaesthesia has been reported. There is no need to change the anaesthetic machine. Continuously flushing the anaesthetic machine and using high fresh gas flow will dry the absorber and is the least useful in solving the problem of CO poisoning.

The following measures should be taken to prevent accidental drying of the CO_2 absorber:

◆ At the end of the list, gas flows should be turned off completely.
◆ If the anaesthetic machine is not used for some time, the CO_2 absorber should be changed irrespective of the change in colour indicator.
◆ If during the weekend, the anaesthetic machine is not used and gas flow is not turned off, the absorber should be changed.

Further reading

1. Coppens MJ, Versichelen LF, Rolly G, *et al.* The mechanism of carbon monoxide production by inhalational agents. *Anaesthesia* 2006; 61: 462-8.
2. Berry PD, Sessler DI, Larson MD. Severe carbon monoxide poisoning during desflurane anesthesia. *Anesthesiology* 1999; 90: 613-6.

29 Answer: B. Size 2.

Choosing an appropriate size of LMA is important to ensure correct positioning and optimal ventilation. A larger mask may cause excessive pressure on the pharyngeal mucosa or may interfere with surgical access in oral surgery. A smaller mask could result in gas leak and inadequate ventilation.

LMA sizes and inflation volumes as recommended by manufacturer are shown in Table 2.

Table 2. LMA sizes and inflation volumes as recommended by manufacturer.

Patient weight (kg)	<5	5-10	10-20	20-30	30-50	50-70	70-100	>100
Size	1	1½	2	2½	3	4	5	6
Maximum inflation volume (ml)	4	7	10	14	20	30	40	50

Further reading

1. Diba A. Airway management devices. In: *Ward's anaesthetic equipment*, 5th ed. Davey AJ, Diba A, Eds. Philadelphia, USA: Elsevier Saunders, 2005; Chapter 8: 165-214.

2. Asai T, Murao K, Yukawa H, Shingu K. Re-evaluation of appropriate size of laryngeal mask airway. *British Journal of Anaesthesia* 1999; 83: 478-9.

3. Brimacombe J, Keller C. Laryngeal mask airway selection in males and females: ease of insertion, oropharyngeal leak pressure, pharyngeal mucosal pressures and anatomical position. *British Journal of Anaesthesia* 1999; 82: 703-7.

30 Answer: A. Evaporation of water from mucus lining the epithelium of the trachea.

During general anaesthesia with tracheal intubation, the upper airway is bypassed and the dry gases from the pipeline are directly delivered to the trachea. The function of the cilia in the mucosal lining of the trachea is to move mucus towards the larynx. Adequate humidity is essential for normal ciliary function. Normally, particles, debris and microbes are trapped in the mucus and are moved towards the larynx and cleared out. Mucus becomes increasingly viscous by breathing dry gases due to the evaporation of water from the mucous lining.

The process of clearance of debris by the movement of mucus towards the larynx is known as the mucociliary elevator mechanism. Loss of this mechanism occurs secondary to evaporation of water from the mucous lining.

The isothermic saturation boundary falls to a lower level within the airway due to heat loss from evaporation. This results in cell damage and infection. In patients who are intubated for several hours or days, thick secretions can block the tracheal tube.

Although breathing dry gases at room temperature contributes to hypothermia, it is not the primary reason for developing respiratory tract infection. It is the evaporation of water from mucus that initiates the cascade of events that ultimately results in infection.

Further reading
1. Wilkes AR. Humidification: its importance and delivery. *British Journal of Anaesthesia CEPD Review* 2001; 1: 40-3.

Set 2 questions

1   A 27-year-old primigravida at 38 weeks' gestation is pre-oxygenated to undergo an emergency Caesarean section under general anaesthesia. Which one of the following physiologic changes mandate pre-oxygenation in this lady?

a.   Reduction in functional residual capacity.
b.   Increase in anatomical dead space.
c.   Increase in minute ventilation.
d.   Increase in the closing capacity.
e.   Increased CO_2 production.

2   A 66-year-old man has an echocardiogram, as part of his pre-operative investigations. The echocardiogram report shows that he has a left ventricular end-diastolic volume of 125ml and end-systolic volume of 50ml. What is his left ventricular ejection fraction?

a.   40%.
b.   50%.
c.   60%.
d.   65%.
e.   55%.

3   A 38-year-old man has had a craniotomy for evacuation of subdural haematoma following a road traffic accident. He has been admitted to intensive care for postoperative management. He has a blood

pressure of 184/92mmHg, his heart rate is 48/minute and his intracranial pressure is 25mmHg. The settings on the ventilator have been altered to deliver high minute ventilation. Which one of the following physiological changes is attributable to the new ventilator setting?

a. Cerebral vasodilatation.
b. Cerebral vasoconstriction.
c. Reduced cerebrospinal fluid pressure.
d. Reduced cerebral oedema.
e. Reduced cerebrospinal fluid production.

4   A 27-year-old woman has had a massive postpartum haemorrhage due to uterine atony. Her haemoglobin is 6g/dL. She has a blood pressure of 106/60mmHg and heart rate of 116/minute. Which one of the following factors most significantly contributes to reduction changes in oxygen delivery to the tissues?

a. Low partial pressure of oxygen.
b. Low arterial oxygen saturation.
c. Low arterial oxygen content.
d. Low mixed venous oxygen saturation.
e. Low cardiac output.

5   A 63-year-old male with a history of atrial fibrillation is usually on warfarin and digoxin. He presents to the emergency department following an overdose of warfarin. Blood results show that his prothrombin time is prolonged. Which of the following combinations of clotting factors could contribute to this abnormal clotting?

a. Clotting Factors II, IV, VIII, IX.
b. Clotting Factors II, VII, IX, X.
c. Clotting Factors VIII, IX, XI, XIII.
d. Clotting Factors II, VIII, X, XII.
e. Clotting Factors II, V, XII, XIII.

6   All volatile anaesthetic agents cause dose-dependent cerebral vasodilatation. Which of the following volatile agents causes the least cerebral vasodilatation?

a.   Isoflurane.
b.   Sevoflurane.
c.   Desflurane.
d.   Halothane.
e.   Enflurane.

7   A 35-year-old male patient with a history of asthma is scheduled for a laparotomy and bowel resection. He is taking 20mg of prednisolone daily. As this patient requires intravenous hydrocortisone during the peri-operative period, which one of the following is equivalent to 20mg prednisolone?

a.   100mg of hydrocortisone.
b.   80mg of hydrocortisone.
c.   75mg of hydrocortisone.
d.   90mg of hydrocortisone.
e.   50mg of hydrocortisone.

8   A 65-year-old woman is brought to the emergency department with major burns. She requires immediate tracheal intubation. Which of the following muscle relaxants is the best choice for rapid sequence induction in this patient?

a.   Rocuronium 0.4mg/kg.
b.   Rocuronium 0.6mg/kg.
c.   Vecuronium 0.1mg/kg.
d.   Atracurium 0.6mg/kg.
e.   Suxamethonium 1mg/kg.

9 A 65-year-old female patient is being assessed in the pre-operative assessment clinic. Her medical history includes hypertension and chronic heart failure. She is already being treated with a diuretic and an ACE inhibitor. Which of the following β-blockers is most suitable to treat her hypertension?

a. Timolol.
b. Propranolol.
c. Labetalol.
d. Esmolol.
e. Bisoprolol.

10 A 5-year-old girl is scheduled for correction of a squint. The pre-operative assessment reveals she is adequately starved but is anxious. The parents state that she gets travel sick. Which one of the following drug combinations is most effective in preventing postoperative nausea and vomiting in this child?

a. Cyclizine 1mg/kg and ondansetron 100μg/kg.
b. Ondansetron 100μg/kg and dexamethasone 100μg/kg.
c. Ondansetron 100μg/kg and dexamethasone 200μg/kg.
d. Cyclizine 1mg/kg and metoclopramide 0.35mg/kg.
e. Ondansetron 100μg/kg alone.

11 When compared to a cylinder manifold, a vacuum-insulated evaporator (VIE) is the most economical way to store and supply oxygen in a large hospital. What is the single most important reason for this?

a. In the long term, it is significantly cheaper to install a VIE.
b. Liquid oxygen is easier to store.
c. VIE does not require rigorous maintenance.
d. When evaporated, liquid oxygen occupies a large volume as gas.
e. The critical temperature of liquid oxygen is ideal to store as a liquid.

12 At the end of an unexpected prolonged procedure for carpal tunnel release under general anaesthesia, it is noted that the patient has developed radial nerve palsy. This persists even at 4 weeks post-procedure. The most likely cause for this is:

a.   Poor patient positioning.
b.   Prolonged application of the tourniquet.
c.   Inappropriately high tourniquet pressure.
d.   Direct trauma due to surgery.
e.   Post-tourniquet syndrome due to interstitial and intracellular oedema.

13 A deep sea SCUBA diver is treated in a hyperbaric chamber for acute decompression sickness. The improvement in symptoms is best explained by:

a.   Dalton's law.
b.   Pascal's principle.
c.   Charles' law.
d.   Henry's law.
e.   Boyle's law.

14 A 4kg infant is admitted for a right inguinal herniotomy. He was born at 28 weeks' gestation. Gas induction was discussed with the parents. What is the fresh gas flow (ml/minute) required to prevent rebreathing with a T-piece circuit?

a.   600ml/ minute.
b.   1000ml/minute.
c.   1600ml/minute.
d.   2400ml/minute.
e.   3000ml/minute.

15 A DC powered operating theatre light produces 96W of energy in the form of heat and light. In order to drive an electric current of 4 amperes through the light bulb, what should be the potential difference across the bulb?

a. 384V.
b. 240V.
c. 96V.
d. 24V.
e. 36V.

16 A 38-year-old man has been admitted to the surgical ward for evaluation of an acute abdomen. On the ward 1L of normal saline has been administered over 30 minutes. This 1L of normal saline will be distributed into the various fluid compartments. Which one of the following statements best describes the distribution of normal saline?

a. 300ml will remain in the intravascular compartment.
b. 500ml will remain in the intravascular compartment.
c. 300ml will be distributed in the extracellular compartment.
d. 500ml will be distributed in the extracellular compartment.
e. 600ml will be distributed to the interstitial fluid compartment.

17 A middle-aged man who has been diagnosed with severe community-acquired pneumonia is being mechanically ventilated in the intensive care unit. The pressure-volume graph obtained on the ventilator is displayed below. Which one of the following physiological attributes is indicated by the inflection points on the above curve?

a. Minute ventilation.
b. Critical opening pressure of the alveoli.
c. Functional residual capacity.
d. Physiological dead space.
e. Expiratory reserve volume.

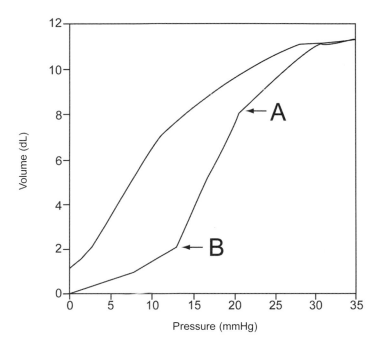

Figure 1. Pressure-volume graph obtained on the ventilator. A = upper inflection point; B = lower inflection point.

18 A 29-year-old female is undergoing laparoscopic gynaecological surgery. The surgeon has requested a head-up position. During the procedure, a rise in arterial pressure is noted. Which one of the following physiologic changes is responsible for the rise in arterial pressure?

a. Increase in stroke volume caused by increased preload.
b. Decrease in heart rate caused by peritoneal stretching.
c. Increase in systemic vascular resistance caused by neurohumoral factors.
d. Increase in intrathoracic pressures caused by pneumoperitoneum.
e. Increase in cardiac output caused by hypercarbia.

19 A 45-year-old male patient who has suffered a spinal cord transection at the C7 level will be unable to control his body temperature when exposed to the operating room temperature of 20°C. What is the most likely reason for this?

a. Inability to sweat.
b. Inability to shiver.
c. Inability to vasoconstrict.
d. Inability to increase cardiac output.
e. Inability to metabolise brown fat.

20 A 65-year-old female patient is admitted to the intensive care unit following a craniotomy and debulking of a posterior fossa tumour. Her serum sodium is 120mmol/L. Which of the following is the most important investigation in establishing the diagnosis of cerebral salt wasting syndrome as a cause of hyponatraemia?

a. Total urinary sodium excretion.
b. Urinary sodium concentration.
c. Serum osmolality.
d. Fractional excretion of uric acid.
e. Urinary osmolality.

21 A 45-year-old male is on morphine sulphate (MST) 50mg b.d., for the management of lower back pain. His pain control is unsatisfactory. Now he has been prescribed buprenorphine 200mg, every 6 hours (in addition to MST). How will this change the efficacy of his morphine?

a. Buprenorphine will enhance the efficacy of morphine.
b. Buprenorphine will reduce the efficacy of morphine.
c. Buprenorphine will not have any effect on morphine efficacy.
d. Buprenorphine will double the efficacy of morphine.
e. Buprenorphine will halve the efficacy of morphine.

22 A 60-year-old male patient is admitted to the intensive care unit with hypotension. His regular medications include amitriptyline 75mg per day and morphine sulphate 100mg per day for chronic back pain. He now needs an inotrope infusion to maintain his blood pressure. Which of the following statements best describes the drug interaction between amitriptyline and inotropes?

a. Amitriptyline potentiates the action of adrenaline more than noradrenaline.
b. Amitriptyline potentiates the action of noradrenaline more than adrenaline.
c. Amitriptyline potentiates the action of both adrenaline and noradrenaline equally.
d. Amitriptyline potentiates the action of only noradrenaline.
e. Amitriptyline potentiates the action of only adrenaline.

23 A 14-month-old child weighing 10kg is scheduled to have bilateral orchidopexy. Which of the following is the most appropriate drug (dose and mixture) for performing caudal anaesthesia in this child?

a. Bupivacaine 0.25% 5ml with clonidine 15µg.
b. Bupivacaine 0.25% 10ml with clonidine 15µg.
c. Bupivacaine 0.5% 10ml with clonidine 15µg.
d. Bupivacaine 0.25% 12.5ml with clonidine 15µg.
e. Bupivacaine 0.25% 12.5ml with adrenaline 1 in 200,000.

24 Which of the following drugs when used for subtenon block has the shortest duration of action?

a. Plain lignocaine.
b. Lignocaine with hyaluronidase.
c. Lignocaine with adrenaline.
d. Lignocaine with bupivacaine.
e. Plain bupivacaine.

25 A newly developed local anaesthetic drug is said to have very high lipid solubility. In practical terms this translates to:

a.   Prolonged duration of action.
b.   Rapid onset of action.
c.   More sensory block than motor block.
d.   Higher potency.
e.   Lower risk of cardiotoxicity.

26 Which of the following best describes the intra-arterial cannula used for the purpose of invasive arterial blood pressure measurement?

a.   It should be short, wide, stiff and with parallel walls.
b.   It should be short, wide, stiff and tapered at the distal end.
c.   It should be short, wide, stiff and transparent.
d.   It should be made of polyurethane.
e.   It should be made of teflon.

27 You are anesthetising a patient for magnetic resonance imaging (MRI). MRI can interfere with the monitoring equipment. Which one of the following best describes the problem of monitoring $EtCO_2$ using side-stream capnography?

a.   The $EtCO_2$ reading is higher than the true value.
b.   The rise time increases.
c.   The transit time increases.
d.   The $EtCO_2$ reading is lower than the true value.
e.   The waveform is distorted.

28 In a cannot intubate, cannot ventilate scenario, the patient should be oxygenated via a cricothyroidotomy. In an adult what is the largest size of tracheostomy tube that can be inserted through the cricothyroid membrane?

a.   Size 8.0.
b.   Size 7.0.

c.   Size 6.0.
d.   Size 5.0.
e.   Size 4.0.

29 A patient is scheduled for an emergency appendicectomy. At the end of an uneventful procedure, a routine check reveals a skin burn at the site of the neutral electrode of the diathermy. The most likely explanation for this injury is:

a.   Delivery of a very high frequency current to coagulate the tissues.
b.   High current density at the site of the neutral electrode.
c.   High impedance at the site of the neutral electrode.
d.   Malfunction of the isolating capacitor.
e.   Use of a floating patient circuit.

30 A Tec 5 isoflurane vaporiser is being used at a high altitude location where the atmospheric pressure is 380mmHg. The dial is set to 1%. The clinical effect on the patient is the same as when using it at sea level (with the dial set to 1%). The most likely reason for this is:

a.   A Tec 5 vaporiser compensates for altitude.
b.   Partial pressure of isoflurane at the alveolus remains the same.
c.   Blood-gas solubility of isoflurane remains the same.
d.   There is no change in the boiling point of isoflurane.
e.   The vapour pressure decreases at high altitude.

Set 2 answers

1 Answer: A. Reduction in functional residual capacity.

Pregnant women are more prone to developing hypoxia following induction of general anaesthesia. In addition to the increased metabolic demands (foetus, placenta and uterus), there are significant changes in the respiratory mechanics that predispose them to hypoxia. Functional residual capacity (FRC) decreases by 20-30% at term due to a reduction of the expiratory reserve volume (by 25%) and residual volume (by 15%). The closing capacity is reduced and can encroach on FRC, resulting in increased ventilation perfusion mismatch.

Dead space is increased by about 40% due to dilatation of large airways; however, the concomitant increase in tidal volume leaves the ratio of dead space to tidal volume unchanged. Minute ventilation is increased by up to 50% above non-pregnant values at term. Since respiratory rate remains unaltered, this increase is due to larger tidal volumes. The increased minute ventilation levels are stimulated by the high progesterone levels and increased CO_2 production occurring during pregnancy. However, the increase in dead space, minute ventilation and CO_2 production do not contribute to increased oxygen requirement.

Further reading
1. Mushambi MC. Physiology of pregnancy. In: *Fundamentals of anaesthesia*, 3rd ed. Pinnock C, Lin T, Smith T, Eds. Cambridge, UK: Cambridge University Press, 2009; Section 2, Chapter 14: 485-98.

2 Answer: C. 60%.

The ejection fraction (EF) is a simple measure of how much of the end-diastolic volume is ejected or pumped out of each ventricle with each contraction. It can be calculated as: (EDV-ESV/EDV) x 100.

The normal values for healthy adult subjects are shown in Table 1.

Table 1. Normal EF values for healthy adult subjects.	
Ejection fraction	60-65%
LV end-systolic volume	40-50ml
LV end-diastolic volume	100-130ml

In heart failure the EF decreases significantly; it can be as low as 20% in severe heart failure. In diastolic dysfunction due to ventricular hypertrophy, EF can be normal despite the presence of ventricular failure. This is because the ventricular filling is impaired due to low ventricular compliance. Both ESV and EDV can be reduced such that EF does not change appreciably. The low ejection fractions are generally associated with systolic dysfunction rather than diastolic dysfunction.

Further reading
1. Swanevelder JLC. Cardiac physiology. In: *Fundamentals of anaesthesia*, 3rd ed. Pinnock C, Lin T, Smith T, Eds. Cambridge, UK: Cambridge University Press, 2009; Chapter 5: 266-96.
2. Rimington H, Chambers J, Eds. Left ventricle. In: *Echocardiography. A practical guide for reporting*, 2nd ed. London, UK: Informa Healthcare, 2007; Chapter 2: 7-9.

3   Answer: B. Cerebral vasoconstriction.

Hyperventilation due to high minute ventilation results in a reduction in partial pressure of carbon dioxide (PCO_2), which reduces hydrogen ions in cerebrospinal fluid (CSF). This causes cerebral vasoconstriction. Maintaining the PCO_2 levels between 4 and 4.5kPa keeps the cerebral blood volume low by preventing vasodilatation and reduces intracranial pressure. However, over 12-24 hours, the buffering mechanism restores pH to normal and vascular tone also returns to its original level.

CSF pressure is not affected by hyperventilation. Hyperventilation-induced vasoconstriction may be helpful in reducing cerebral oedema.

The mainstay of management in this patient would be to prevent secondary brain injury which can be caused by hypoxia, hypotension, hypercarbia, hyperthermia and hyperglycaemia. In addition to hyperventilation, other non-pharmacological methods of controlling intracranial pressure are to maintain head elevation, hypothermia, drainage of cerebrospinal fluid (e.g. external ventricular drain) and decompressive surgery.

Further reading
1. Menon DK, Eynon CA. Critical care management of head injury. *Anaesthesia and Intensive Care Medicine* 2002; 2: 135-9.
2. Turner JM, Menon DK, Matta BF, Eds. Pathophysiology, initial resuscitation and transfer. In: *Textbook of neuroanaesthesia and critical care*. London, UK: Greenwich Medical Media, 2000; Section 5, Chapter 20: 285-99.
3. Roberts I, Scierhout G. Hyperventilation therapy for acute traumatic brain injury. http://www2.cochrane.org/reviews/en/ab000566.html.

4 Answer: C. Low arterial oxygen content.

The oxygen content of the blood depends on oxygen saturation and haemoglobin in the blood, and can be calculated from the following equation:

$$\text{Arterial oxygen content (ml/dL)} = \frac{\text{Hb} \times 1.34 \times \text{SaO}_2\,(\%)}{100} + (0.003 \times \text{PaO}_2)$$

Where Hb = haemoglobin; SaO_2 = percentage of haemoglobin saturated with oxygen; PaO_2 = partial pressure of arterial oxygen in mm Hg.

1g of haemoglobin can carry 1.34ml of oxygen if fully saturated.

Oxygen delivery to the tissues is calculated by multiplying cardiac output (CO) and arterial oxygen content (CaO_2) of the blood.

As this patient has a low haemoglobin, oxygen delivery to the tissues is reduced due to low oxygen content of the arterial blood. The compensatory response to acute anaemia would be an increase in cardiac output, predominantly by an increase in the heart rate, in order to maintain adequate tissue perfusion and oxygen delivery.

At a PO_2 of 13.3kPa (100mmHg), Hb is normally about 98% saturated with oxygen. If the Hb is 15g/100ml, arterial blood will carry 200ml/dL of oxygen. With a cardiac output of 5L/minute, the amount of oxygen available in the circulation is 1000ml/minute. Of this, approximately 250ml/minute is used at rest, the Hb in venous blood being about 75% saturated.

PaO_2 is a measurement of pressure exerted by oxygen molecules dissolved in plasma; once oxygen molecules chemically bind to haemoglobin they no longer exert any pressure. Although factors such as anaemia, carbon monoxide poisoning, methemoglobinaemia will reduce the oxygen delivery to the tissues, they do not affect PaO_2. Oxygen saturation remains normal in anaemia, unless the gas exchange is impaired due to ventilation perfusion mismatch from a low cardiac output.

Mixed venous oxygen saturation (SVO_2) is the O_2 saturation of blood in the pulmonary artery. It is related to arterial oxygen content, oxygen consumption and cardiac output. Normal values being 75%, oxygen delivery is considered critical at values lower than 50%. In patients with acute anaemia, the reduction in arterial content is counterbalanced by a compensatory increase in cardiac output which maintains the mixed venous oxygen saturation levels close to normal values.

The compensatory response to acute anaemia would be an increase in cardiac output, predominantly by an increase in the heart rate, in order to maintain adequate tissue perfusion and oxygen delivery. However, if there is continuing blood loss, the cardiac output would reduce, leading to haemorrhagic shock.

Further reading
1. Appadu BL, Hanning CD. Respiratory physiology. In: *Fundamentals of anaesthesia*, 3rd ed. Pinnock C, Lin T, Smith T, Eds. Cambridge, UK: Cambridge University Press, 2009; Section 2, Chapter 8: 373-5.

5   Answer: B. Clotting Factors II, VII, IX, X.

Clotting Factors II, VII, IX and X are synthesised in the liver. They are biologically inactive unless 9 to 13 of the amino-terminal glutamate residues are carboxylated to form the Ca^{2+}-binding g-carboxyglutamate residues. This reaction requires CO_2, molecular oxygen, reduced vitamin K and is catalysed by g-glutamyl carboxylase. Carboxylation is directly coupled to the oxidation of vitamin K to its corresponding epoxide. Reduced vitamin K must be regenerated from the epoxide for sustained carboxylation and synthesis of biologically competent proteins. The enzyme that catalyzes this, vitamin K epoxide reductase, is inhibited by therapeutic doses of warfarin.

Oral anticoagulants have no effect on the activity of fully carboxylated molecules in the circulation. Thus, the time required for the activity of each factor in plasma to reach a new steady state after therapy is initiated or adjusted, depends on its individual rate of clearance.

The above clotting factors have a variable half-life (Table 2).

Table 2. Clotting factors and half-lives.	
Clotting Factor	**Half-life**
Clotting Factor VII	6 hours
Clotting Factor IX	24 hours
Clotting Factor X	36 hours
Clotting Factor II	50 hours

Because of the long half-lives of some of the coagulation factors, in particular Factor II, the full antithrombotic effect of warfarin is not achieved for several days, even though the prothrombin time may be prolonged soon after administration due to the more rapid reduction of factors with a shorter half-life, in particular Factor VII.

Further reading
1. Ganong WF, Ed. Haemostasis. In: *Review of medical physiology*, 22nd ed. New York, USA: McGraw-Hill, 2005; Section 6, Chapter 27: 540-6.
2. Majerus PW, Tollefsen DM. Blood coagulation and anticoagulant, thrombolytic and antiplatelet drugs. In: *Goodman and Gilman's - the pharmacological basis of therapeutics*, 11th ed. New York, USA: McGraw-Hill, 2006; Section 11, Chapter 54: 1467-88.

6   Answer: B. Sevoflurane.

All volatile anaesthetic agents increase cerebral blood flow (CBF) and can result in a dose-dependent increase in intracranial pressure. The order of vasodilating potency is halothane >enflurane >desflurane >isoflurane >sevoflurane.

All volatile anaesthetic agents have a direct effect on the vascular smooth muscle. But the overall effect on cerebral blood flow depends on several other factors such as partial pressure of CO_2, the MAC of the anaesthetic agent, changes in blood pressure and pre-existing abnormality with autoregulation.

Halothane at 1 MAC, has shown to increase CBF significantly. Enflurane increases CBF at 1.2 MAC. Both agents result in a modest reduction in cerebral metabolic rate (CMR). The effect of isoflurane on CBF is much less than halothane and enflurane.

Further reading
1. Drummond JC, Patel PM. Neurosurgical anaesthesia. In: *Miller's anesthesia,* Volume 1, 7th ed. Miller RD, Ed. Philadelphia, USA: Churchill Livingstone, 2010; Chapter 25: 2048-9.

7 Answer: B. 80mg of hydrocortisone.

5mg of prednisolone is equivalent to 20mg of hydrocortisone. Therefore, 20mg prednisolone is equivalent to 80mg of hydrocortisone.

The relative potencies of steroid preparation are shown in Table 3.

Table 3. Relative potencies of steroid preparation.	
Dexamethasone	1
Methylprednisolone	4
Prednisolone	5
Hydrocortisone	20
Cortisone acetate	25

Further reading
1. Nicholson G, Burrin JM, Hall GM. Peri-operative steroid supplementation. *Anaesthesia* 1998; 53: 1091-104

8   Answer: E. Suxamethonium 1mg/kg.

Suxamethonium provides a rapid onset of depolarizing neuromuscular block with best intubating conditions even when compared to rocuronium. Although hyperkalaemia is a recognized complication in patients with burns, it does not occur in the first 24 hours, and usually occurs 1 to 10 weeks following burns. This is due to proliferation of extra-junctional receptors. Rocuronium is the second best choice for rapid sequence induction when administered at a dose of 0.9mg/kg.

Depolarisation of the motor endplate and muscle contraction causes the efflux of potassium ions into the extracellular fluid. Usually this increases serum potassium by about 0.5mmol/L and does not have any clinical significance. In patients with burns and neurological diseases, an abnormal hyperkalaemic response may be seen, with a massive increase in serum potassium levels resulting in hyperkalaemic cardiac arrest.

Further reading
1. Perry JJ, Lee JS, Sillberg VA, Wells GA. Rocuronium versus succinylcholine for rapid sequence induction intubation. *Cochrane Database Syst Rev* 2008; CD002788.

9   Answer: E. Bisoprolol.

Bisoprolol is a β1 selective anatagonist. The CIBIS-II (Cardiac Insufficiency Bisoprolol Study-II) trial has shown a significant reduction in the rate of sudden deaths and reduction in pump failure in patients treated with bisoprolol. The actual mechanism of benefit of β-blockers in heart failure is not fully understood. The most likely mechanism is that they decrease the incidence of malignant ventricular arrhythmias. It also improves left ventricular function.

Timolol is a non-selective β-blocker used in hypertension, angina and the prophylaxis of migraine. Propranolol is also a non-selective β-blocker used in thyrotoxicosis, angina and the prophylaxis of migraine. Labetalol has both α and β effects (β-block is seven times greater than α-block when administered IV and three times greater than α-block when administered orally). It is used in the treatment of angina and hypertension.

Esmolol is a cardioselective β-blocker with a rapid onset and offset of action. Therefore, it is mainly used in the short-term management of tachycardia, hypertension and acute supraventricular tachycardia. It is administered as an IV bolus followed by an IV infusion.

Further reading
1. McGavin JK, Keating GM. Bisoprolol: a review in chronic heart failure. *Drugs* 2002; 62: 2677-96.
2. The cardiac insufficiency bisoprolol study II (CIBIS-II): a randomized trial. *Lancet* 1999; 353: 9-13.

10 Answer: B. Ondansetron 100µg/kg and dexamethasone 100µg/kg.

A combination of two drugs is more likely to be effective in reducing the incidence of postoperative nausea and vomiting (PONV), when compared to a single drug. Cyclizine is not used in children younger than 6 years. Metoclopramide is a prokinetic drug and is not effective in the prevention of nausea and vomiting. 5-HT3 receptor agonists such as ondansetron and dexamethasone are commonly used in children for the prevention of nausea and vomiting. Dexamethasone at a dose of 100µg/kg has been found to be as effective as higher doses in the prophylaxis of PONV.

Further reading
1. APAGBI guidelines 2009. Guidelines on the prevention of postoperative nausea and vomiting in children. http://www.apagbi.org.uk/sites/apagbi.org.uk/files/APA_Guidelines_ on_the_Prevention_of_Postoperative_Vomiting_in_Children.pdf.
2. Gan TJ, Meyer T, Apfel CC. Consensus guidelines for managing postoperative nausea and vomiting. *Anesthesia and Analgesia* 2003; 97: 62-71.

11 Answer: D. When evaporated, liquid oxygen occupies a large volume as gas.

Liquid oxygen is stored in a vacuum-insulated evaporator (VIE) at a temperature of -150°C to -170°C and at a pressure of 5-10 atmospheres. In simple terms this works like a giant thermos flask. At 15°C, one volume of liquid oxygen occupies 842 times its volume as gas. Oxygen constantly evaporates from the top of the VIE. As this oxygen is very cold, it needs to be passed through a super heater. When the oxygen flows at a faster rate, the temperature of the liquid falls due to the latent heat of evaporation. To overcome this problem additional heat is provided by a pressure-raising vaporiser.

Regular maintenance, monitoring of usage of oxygen and topping up the tank at regular intervals is necessary.

Further reading
1. Al-Shaikh B, Stacey S, Eds. Liquid oxygen. In: *Essentials of anaesthetic equipment*, 3rd ed. London, UK: Churchill Livingstone, Elsevier, 2007; Chapter 1: 9-10.

12 Answer: C. Inappropriately high tourniquet pressure.

Tissue compression due to high tourniquet pressure predominantly affects nerve tissue. A physiological conduction block develops about 15 and 45 minutes after inflation of a cuff around the arm, to a pressure above systolic pressure. This is reversible at the end of the procedure. In contrast, high cuff pressures result in morphological changes within the larger myelinated nerves. These include displacement of the nodes of Ranvier, stretching and degeneration of paranodal myelin. The impaired nerve conduction may last up to 6 months.

Poor patient positioning can result in nerve injury. The ulnar nerve at the elbow is more susceptible to compression between the bone and hard surface.

Muscle ischaemia due to the tourniquet results in a progressive decrease in PO_2 and an increase in PCO_2 and lactate within muscle cells. Marked changes in mitochondrial morphology are visible after an hour of ischaemia. Once the tourniquet is released, increased vascular permeability results in interstitial and intracellular oedema. This leads to the post-tourniquet syndrome, in which the patient has a swollen, pale, stiff limb with weakness but no paralysis. This may last for 1-6 weeks.

Further reading
1. Deloughry JL, Griffiths R. Arterial tourniquets. *British Journal of Anaesthesia CEACCP* 2009; 9: 56-61.

13 Answer: E. Boyle's law.

At depth, the diver is subjected to a high atmospheric pressure. During this phase, nitrogen is dissolved in the tissues. On rapid ascent to sea level, the dissolved gas precipitates as bubbles. These bubbles can mechanically obstruct the tissue and cause disruption of cells. This is the initial event in decompression sickness.

Boyle's law states that at constant temperature, the volume of a gas varies inversely with the pressure. Treatment for acute decompression sickness is recompression in a hyperbaric chamber. This reduces the size of air bubbles.

Dalton's law explains the physiological effects of gases: the partial pressure of a gas in a mixture is proportional to its percentage by volume in the mixture. It is equal to the fractional concentration multiplied by ambient pressure (which is proportional to depth).

Pascal's principle is that pressure applied to a liquid will be transmitted equally throughout the liquid. Gases are compressible and fluids are relatively incompressible. The human body is mainly composed of water and so the pressure is transmitted evenly throughout the body, as predicted by Pascal's principle, until it meets a gas-containing cavity. If the walls of the cavity are distensible, the cavity will change in volume as predicted by Boyle's law.

Henry's law explains the solubility of gases in fluids. It states that at constant temperature, the volume of gas dissolved in solution in a given liquid is proportional to the partial pressure of the gas.

Further reading
1. Williams DJ. Bubble trouble: an introduction to diving medicine. *British Journal of Anaesthesia CEACCP* 2002; 2: 144-7.

14   Answer: D. 2400ml/minute.

This child weighs 4kg. The tidal volume required is 10ml per kg of body weight. Minute volume is tidal volume x respiratory rate. In an infant, the respiratory rate is around 20 breaths per minute.

A T-piece system requires a fresh gas flow of 2.5 to 3 times the minute volume to prevent rebreathing.

This child requires 40ml of tidal volume. So the minute volume is 800ml.

Minimum gas flow = 800 x 2.5-3 = 2000-2400ml/minute.

The T-piece is a valveless breathing system, particularly used in children weighing up to 25-30kg. It is suitable for both spontaneous and controlled ventilation. It comprises a T-shaped tubing with three ports: the first port for fresh gas flow, the second port goes to the patient and the third port connects to the reservoir tubing. The system requires a fresh gas flow of 2.5 to 3 times the minute volume to prevent rebreathing with a minimal flow of 4L/minute. It requires a high fresh gas flow during spontaneous ventilation. Since there is no APL valve in this breathing system, scavenging is a problem.

Further reading
1. Al-Shaikh B, Stacey S. T-piece system. In: *Essentials of anaesthetic equipment*, 3rd ed. Parkinson M. London, UK: Churchill Livingstone, Elsevier, 2007; Chapter 4: 53-4.

15 Answer: D. 24V.

The potential difference can be calculated using the following formula:

$$\text{Potential difference (V)} = \text{Power (Watt)}/\text{Current (A)}$$
$$\text{In this scenario, } V = 96/4 = 24V$$

The potential difference in volts = Power in Watts/Current in amperes.

One volt is the difference of electrical potential between two points of a conductor carrying a constant current of 1 ampere, when the power dissipated between these points is 1 Watt.

Power is the rate of energy expenditure. One Watt is one Joule/second.

Further reading
1. Davis PD, Kenny GNC. Heat production and AC units. In: *Basic physics and measurement in anaesthesia*, 5th ed. London, UK; Butterworth Heinemann, 2003; Chapter 14: 153.

16 Answer: A. 300ml will remain in the intravascular compartment.

Total body water (TBW) can be divided into intracellular fluid (ICF) and extracellular fluid (ECF) compartments. ICF comprises about 2/3 (66%) and ECF comprises 1/3 (33%) of TBW. Approximately 60% of ECF is comprised of interstitial fluid, whilst 30% is comprised of intravascular compartments.

A 0.9% solution of NaCl (normal saline) is nearly isotonic. Therefore, it distributes equally in the ECF compartment. Following intravenous administration of 1L of normal saline (assuming no capillary leak and normal osmotic forces), approximately 30% of the fluid would remain in the intravascular compartment while the rest of the fluid would be distributed to other extracellular compartments (interstitial and transcellular compartments).

The sodium in normal saline would not be distributed into the intracellular fluid compartment, as the cell membrane is not permeable to sodium. Sodium transport across the cell membrane is regulated by the sodium-potassium pumps on the cell membrane. Hence, normal saline is distributed only in the extracellular fluid compartment.

Further reading
1. Ganong WF, Ed. Regulation of extracellular fluid composition and volume. In: *Review of medical physiology*, 22nd ed. New York, USA: McGraw-Hill, 2005; Section 8, Chapter 39: 729-30.

17 Answer: B. Critical opening pressure of the alveoli.

The curve describes the relationship between volume and pressure. The ideal level of PEEP is that which puts the majority of lung units on the favourable part of the pressure-volume curve, maximizes gas exchange and minimizes over-distension. The pressure-volume curve helps to

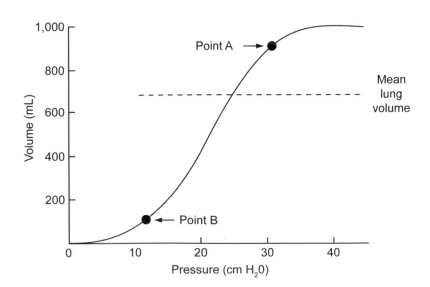

Figure 1. Pressure volume curve. A = upper inflection point; B = lower inflection point.

determine the critical opening pressure for the majority of alveoli (the lower inflection point). At this point, the majority of the collapsed alveoli open and the lung becomes more compliant. With further increases in pressure, the lung volume increases linearly with increasing pressure until it reaches the upper inflection point. At this point, the pressure-volume curve flattens and any ventilation with a pressure higher than this could damage the lung.

Respiratory volume measurements can be made using spirometry. Minute ventilation can be calculated from tidal volumes and respiratory rate.

Functional residual capacity is the sum of expiratory reserve volume and residual volume (RV). FRC can be measured uisng nitrogen washout helium dilution or body plethysmography. It cannot be measured using spirometry.

Physiological dead space is anatomical plus alveolar dead space, which can be measured using the Bohr equation.

Further reading
1. Allen GB, Parsons PE. Acute respiratory failure due to ARDS and pulmonary edema. In: *Irwin and Rippe's intensive care medicine*, 6th ed. Irwin RS, Rippe JM, Eds. Philadelphia, USA: Lippincott Williams & Wilkins, 2008; Section 4, Chapter 46: 502-5.

18 Answer: C. Increase in systemic vascular resistance caused by neurohumoral factors.

Systemic vascular resistance is a major contributor in maintaining blood pressure during laparoscopic procedures involving pneumoperitoneum. The release of neurohumoral factors such as vasopressin and catecholamines causes a rise in systemic vascular resistance.

Carbon dioxide absorption from the peritoneal cavity causes hypercarbia which in turn stimulates the release of catecholamines contributing to a rise in systemic vascular resistance. The return of hemodynamic parameters to baseline values is gradual, taking several minutes, suggesting the involvement of neurohumoral factors.

Mechanical stimulation of peritoneal receptors also results in increased vasopressin release. The increase in systemic vascular resistance is affected by patient position. The Trendelenburg position attenuates the increase while the head-up position aggravates it.

Peritoneal stretch caused by gas insufflation stimulates the vagal nerve resulting in a decrease in heart rate. Heart rate increases slowly due to neurohumoral stimulation caused by the surgical stress and hypercarbia.

Peritoneal insufflation of gas causes a rise in intra-abdominal pressure pushing the diaphragm upwards resulting in a rise in intrathoracic pressure. This is further increased in the Trendelenberg position.

Increased intra-abdominal pressure decreases venous return. When intra-abdominal pressure is higher than inferior vena cava pressure, venous return decreases and results in pooling of blood in the legs and an increase in venous resistance.

Hypercarbia at the cellular level causes depression of myocardial contractility and the rate of contraction but increases the irritability and arrhythmogenicity of the myocardium. It causes peripheral vasodilatation. It also causes profound systemic changes secondary to sympathoadrenal and central nervous system stimulation.

Further reading
1. Joris JL. Anesthesia for laparoscopic surgery. In: *Miller's anesthesia*, Volume 2, 7th ed. Miller RD, Ed. Philadelphia, USA: Churchill Livingstone, Elsevier, 2010; Chapter 68: 2189-90.

19   Answer: C. Inability to vasoconstrict.

When the environmental temperature is less than body temperature, the body loses heat by conduction and radiation. Conduction is aided by convection where the molecules move away from the area of contact. In the operating room, this accounts for a small fraction of total heat loss. The amount of heat loss by conduction depends on skin temperature. The amount of heat reaching the skin depends on blood flow to the skin.

Any object that has a temperature above absolute zero emits infra-red rays. Radiation accounts for the majority of heat loss (>60%). The amount of heat lost by radiation is influenced by skin blood flow. Water evaporation and sweating results in heat loss. For each gram of water that is evaporated, 0.58kcal of heat is lost.

The mechanisms that reduce heat loss include cutaneous vasoconstriction, change of position (curling up) to reduce the surface area and horripilation (goose bumps - mediated by noradrenergic $\alpha1$ receptors).

The mechanisms that increase heat production include increased voluntary activity and shivering. Brown fat metabolism increases heat production; this mechanism is only seen in infants.

Further reading
1. Ganong WF, Ed. Temperature regulation. In: *Review of medical physiology*, 22nd ed. New York, USA: McGraw-Hill, 2005; Section 3, Chapter 14: 251-5.

20 Answer: A. Total urinary sodium excretion.

The most common cause of hyponatraemia is the syndrome of inappropriate ADH secretion (SIADH). Cerebral salt wasting syndrome (CSWS) also causes hyponatraemia, and is seen in patients with traumatic brain injury.

Urinary sodium concentration is elevated in both SIADH and cerebral salt wasting syndrome (>40mmol/L). However, total urinary sodium excretion (urine sodium concentration x urine volume in 24 hours) is substantially higher than sodium intake in cerebral salt wasting syndrome but generally equals sodium intake in SIADH. Therefore, the net sodium balance (intake minus output) is negative in cerebral salt wasting syndrome.

Fractional excretion of uric acid (FEUA) is defined as the percentage of urate filtered by the glomeruli that is excreted in urine. Patients with either cerebral salt wasting syndrome or SIADH can have hypouricaemia and elevated FEUA. However, after correction of hyponatraemia, hypouricaemia and elevated FEUA may normalize in SIADH but persist in cerebral salt wasting syndrome. Serum osmolality is reduced in both SIADH and CSWS. Urinary osmolality is increased in both of these conditions.

Excessive renal excretion of sodium leads to depletion of extracellular volume and reduced effective circulating volume. Reduced circulating volume and reduced blood pressure activates baroreceptors which increases the secretion of antidiuretic hormone from the posterior pituitary. This leads to water retention and restores the extracellular fluid volume.

Failure to distinguish CSWS from SIADH as the cause of hyponatraemia could lead to inappropriate therapy (i.e. fluid restriction). This can exacerbate extracellular volume depletion and compromise cerebral perfusion.

The possible mechanism is that the injured brain may release natriuretic proteins that act directly on the renal tubules. In addition, cerebral injury may increase sympathetic nervous system activity, elevating renal perfusion pressure and releasing dopamine.

Further reading
1. Springate JE, Garimella-Krovi S. Cerebral salt wasting syndrome. http://emedicine.medscape.com/article/919609.

21 Answer: B. Buprenorphine will reduce the efficacy of morphine.

Buprenorphine is a partial agonist at μ receptors and morphine is a full agonist at the same receptors. Buprenorphine will occupy some of the μ receptors without exerting maximum efficacy, thus it will reduce the number of receptors available for morphine, which has maximum efficacy at μ receptors. Therefore, the efficacy of morphine will decrease. The reduction in efficacy depends on the doses of full agonist and partial agonist and it is difficult to predict the precise reduction in efficacy from the information available in this scenario.

Further reading
1. Calvey TN, Williams NE. Drug action. In: *Principles and practice of pharmacology for anaesthetists*, 4th ed. Oxford, UK: Blackwell Science, 2001; Chapter 3: 57-8.

22 Answer: B. Amitriptyline potentiates the action of noradrenaline more than adrenaline.

Noradrenaline is partly removed from the synaptic cleft by active transport back into the nerve terminal. This mechanism can be blocked by most tricyclic antidepressants and their derivatives, which compete with catecholamines for axonal transport. The pressor response to noradrenaline is potentiated 4-9 times in the presence of these agents, while the effect of adrenaline is increased only by 2-3 times.

Further reading
1. Calvey TN, Williams NE. Drug interaction. In: *Principles and practice of pharmacology for anaesthetists*, 4th ed. Oxford, UK: Blackwell Science, 2001; Chapter 4: 74-6.

63

23 Answer: B. Bupivacaine 0.25% 10ml with clonidine 15µg.

Caudal anaesthesia is the most frequently used technique of paediatric regional anaesthesia. The volume of local anaesthetics used depends on the level of block required and the total recommended dose. The recommended doses of local anaesthetic are shown in Table 4.

Table 4. Recommended doses of local anaesthetic.	
Level of block	**Volume of local anaesthetic required**
Sacral	0.5ml/kg 0.25% bupivacaine
Lumbar	1ml/kg 0.25% bupivacaine
Thoraco-lumbar	1.25ml/kg 0.19% bupivacaine

Drugs such as ketamine (0.5mg/kg), clonidine 1-2µg/kg, diamorphine (30µg/kg) or morphine (50µg/kg) can be added to extend the duration of block. Adrenaline has been reported to cause spinal ischaemia and should be avoided.

Further reading
1. Allman KG, Wilson IH. Paediatric and neonatal anaesthesia. In: *Oxford handbook of anaesthesia*, 2nd ed. Oxford, UK: Oxford University Press, 2006; Chapter 33: 784-7.

24   Answer: B. Lignocaine with hyaluronidase.

Hyaluronidase is an enzyme used to enhance permeation of injected fluids or local anaesthetics. The addition of hyaluronidase to local anaesthetic solutions may significantly reduce the duration of blockade. The addition of adrenaline to local anaesthetic prolongs the duration of action. Adrenaline causes vasoconstriction and reduces the absorption of local anaesthetic from the injected site.

Further reading
1. Calvey TN, Williams NE. Drug interaction. In: *Principles and practice of pharmacology for anaesthetists*, 4th ed. Oxford, UK: Blackwell Science, 2001; Chapter 4: 74-6.

25   Answer: D. Higher potency.

There is a close correlation between lipid solubility and anaesthetic potency especially in *in vitro* conditions. This reflects the ability of the drug to penetrate perineural tissues and the neuronal membrane, and reach their site of action in the axoplasm.

Tissue protein binding primarily affects the duration of action of local anaesthetics, whereas speed of onset is determined by the dissociation constant (pKa). The amount of ionised drug depends on the pKa of that drug and pH of the surrounding tissue. Only the unionised form of the local anaesthetic diffuses through the lipid layer (neuronal membrane). But the ionised form of local anaesthetic is the active form that blocks sodium channels and produces the clinical effect. Lignocaine has a pKa of 7.9 and is about 25% unionised at a pH of 7.4. Bupivacaine has a pKa of 8.1 and is about 15% unionised at a pH of 7.4. Therefore, when compared to bupivacaine, a larger proportion of lignocaine passes through the lipid cell membrane.

Further reading
1. Calvey TN, Williams NE. Local anaesthetics. In: *Principles and practice of pharmacology for anaesthetists*, 4th ed. Oxford, UK: Blackwell Science, 2001; Chapter 8: 154-7.

26 Answer: A. It should be short, wide, stiff and with parallel walls.

The diameter of the cannula used to cannulate the artery is a balance between a small cannula (22 or 20 gauge) that carries a lower incidence of thrombus formation and a larger catheter (18 or 16 gauge) that is less likely to kink or become blocked. Arterial cannulae are made of teflon or polyurethane and have parallel walls to minimize the effect on blood flow to the distal part of the limb. A short, wide, stiff and parallel-sided catheter is useful in minimising the effects on the resonant frequency of the system.

Further reading
1. Al-Shaikh B, Stacey S, Eds. Invasive monitoring. In: *Essentials of anaesthetic equipment*, 3rd ed. London, UK: Churchill Livingstone, Elsevier, 2007; Chapter 11: 162-3.
2. Davis PD, Kenny GNC. Blood pressure measurement. In: *Basic physics and measurement in anaesthesia*, 5th ed. London, UK: Butterworth-Heinemann, 2003; Chapter 17: 192-3.

27 Answer: C. The transit time increases.

The most significant problem associated with magnetic resonance imaging (MRI) is the attraction of ferromagnetic objects to the magnetic field. The displays on standard monitors can be distorted by the magnetic field and the monitors themselves can degrade the MRI image by altering the signal/noise ratio.

The transit time is the time required for the sample to move from the point of sampling to the detector cell. In the MRI suite the side-stream analyser should be kept away from the magnetic field. Therefore, a long sampling tube is required. This prolongs the transit time. A prolonged transit time delays the appearance of the waveform at the monitor resulting in phase shift but no distortion. The actual $EtCO_2$ reading is not affected.

The rise time is the time taken by the output from the capnometer to change from 10% of final value to the 90% final value in response to a step change in partial pressure of CO_2. It is dependent on the size of the sample chamber and the gas flow rate.

The response time is the combination of rise time and transit time. A response time less than one respiratory cycle is ideal.

Further reading
1. Bhavani-Shankar K. Capnometry and anaesthesia. *Canadian Journal of Anaesthesia* 1992; 39: 617-32.
2. Peden CJ, Twigg SJ. Anaesthesia for magnetic resonance imaging. *British Journal of Anaesthesia CEPD review* 2003; 3: 97-101.

28 Answer: C. Size 6.0.

The cricothyroid (CT) membrane is the first indentation felt in the midline, inferior to the thyroid cartilage. It is a dense fibro-elastic, relatively avascular and relatively superficial membrane bordered laterally by cricothyroid muscles.

The width of the CT membrane varies between 22-33mm in adults and the height between 9-10mm. The outer diameter of the endotracheal tube should therefore not exceed 9mm. A tracheostomy tube with a 6mm internal diameter has an outer diameter of 8.3mm (Portex blue line cuffed tube). Therefore, size 6.0 is the largest tracheostomy tube that can be used for a surgical cricothyroidotomy in adults.

Further reading
1. Boon JM, Abrahams PH, *et al.* Cricothyroidotomy: a clinical anatomy review. *Clinical Anatomy* 2004; 17: 478-86.

29 Answer: B. High current density at the site of the neutral electrode.

Poor contact between the skin and the neutral electrode results in high current density at the site of the neutral electrode. This results in excessive heating and skin burns. The conducting and contractile tissues are maximally sensitive to electric current at the mains frequency of 50Hz. Diathermy uses a very high frequency current (0.5-1.5MHz) to coagulate the tissue. This high frequency current does not cause excitation of contractile tissues.

Partial or intermittent contact of the neutral plate with the skin results in areas of high current density. The amount of heat generated is proportional to the square of current divided by the area.

$$H = I^2/A$$

Where H = heat generated; I = current; and A = area.

At the tip of the diathermy forceps a lot of heat is generated due to the small area of contact. The neutral electrode (patient's plate) has a large surface area, and when correctly placed, produces no heat due to a very low current density.

Further reading
1. Al-Shaikh B, Stacey S. Electrical safety. In: *Essentials of anaesthetic equipment*, 3rd ed. London, UK: Churchill Livingstone, Elsevier, 2007; Chapter 14: 211-23.

30 Answer: B. Partial pressure of isoflurane at the alveolus remains the same.

At high altitude the atmospheric pressure decreases. The saturated vapour pressure (SVP) of isoflurane does not change (SVP changes with change in temperature not with change in atmospheric pressure). The concentration delivered by the vaporiser increases because SVP takes up a high proportion of ambient pressure. Hence, at any given dial setting the delivered percentage of inhalational agents will increase with altitude (decrease in barometric pressure); however, its partial pressure will remain constant.

The clinical effect of isoflurane is determined by the alveolar partial pressure rather than the concentration delivered by the vaporiser. The partial pressure of isoflurane at the alveolus remains constant. This reflects the partial pressure of isoflurane in the brain. The vaporiser dial setting should remain constant irrespective of altitude to produce the same clinical effect.

Further reading

1. Carter JA. Provision of anaesthesia in difficult situations and the developing world. In: *Ward's anaesthetic equipment*, 5th ed. Davey AJ, Diba A, Eds. Philadelphia, USA: Elsevier Saunders, 2005; Chapter 29: 485-98.
2. Roy PK. Physiological adaptation and anaesthesia at high altitude. *Indian Journal of Anaesthesia* 2002; 46: 175-81.

Set 3 questions

1 A 32-year-old lady, who is known to have type 1 diabetes mellitus, presents to the accident and emergency department with reduced consciousness and deep shallow breathing. Her blood results are shown in Table 1.

Table 1. Blood results.			
Sodium	136mmol/L	pH	7.2
Potassium	4.0mmol/L	PO_2	13.2kPa
Chloride	102mmol/L	PCO_2	2.9kPa
Magnesium	0.8mmol/L	HCO_3^-	12mmol/L
Blood glucose	34.8mmol/L	Base excess	-14.0mmol/L

Which one of the following most accurately indicates the anion gap value in this patient?

a. 24mmol/L.
b. 20mmol/L.
c. 26mmol/L.
d. 8mmol/L.
e. 18mmol/L.

2   You are part of the obstetric and paediatric team at Lhasa, Tibet (altitude - 10,000ft). You attend a newborn resuscitation call, for a baby who is born at 39 weeks' gestation, a normal delivery. The mother has no medical problems and the baby has no obvious congenital anomalies. Which one of the following cardiac physiological changes is more likely to occur in this baby?

a.   Low right atrial pressure.
b.   High pulmonary artery pressure.
c.   Higher than normal heart rate.
d.   High systemic vascular resistance.
e.   High stroke volume.

3   A 5-year-old child is scheduled to undergo a complex surgical procedure on the forearm. The child weighs 20kg. The blood results are: Hb: 13g/dL, PCV: 40%, platelets: 392 x10^9/L. The plastic surgeon prefers to maintain haematocrit levels at 30% for the first 24-48 hours in the postoperative period. Assuming the blood volume to be 70ml/kg, what would be the maximum allowable blood loss for this child?

a.   450ml.
b.   350ml.
c.   250ml.
d.   500ml.
e.   175ml.

4   A 46-year-old man was found unconscious at home and is brought to the emergency department by the paramedics. His blood gases show that he is acidotic. He is suspected to have starved for almost a week. Which of the following biochemical changes is most likely to present in his blood?

a.   Low blood glucose levels.
b.   Reduced protein breakdown.

c.   Increased free fatty acids.
d.   Low levels of ketones.
e.   Low levels of magnesium.

5   A 63-year-old male who is scheduled for a bowel resection is seen
     in the pre-operative assessment clinic. He has smoked 20 cigarettes
     a day for more than 30 years. Which one of the following
     physiological changes is most likely to occur in this patient as
     compared to a non-smoker?

a.   Shift to the right of the oxygen dissociation curve.
b.   Reduced FEV1.
c.   Reduced closing capacity.
d.   Low airway resistance.
e.   Increase in FVC.

6   Concurrent administration of midazolam 5mg and propofol 150mg,
     intravenously, in a 60-year-old male produces a significant hypnotic
     effect which is greater than the expected combined effect of the two
     drugs. This phenomenon is best described by:

a.   Summation.
b.   Potentiation.
c.   Agonistic action.
d.   Synergism.
e.   Antagonism.

7   A 63-year-old male is due to undergo an emergency laparotomy for
     bowel obstruction. He takes selegiline for Parkinson's disease.
     Which one of the following analgesics is safe and appropriate to use
     in this patient for postoperative pain relief?

a.   Pethidine.
b.   Morphine.
c.   Methadone.
d.   Tramadol.
e.   Remifentanil.

8 Acute hepatic porphyria is a rare but significant complication, which can occur after administration of certain anaesthetic drugs in a patient with a deficiency of α levulinic acid synthetase enzyme. Which one of the following terms most appropriately explains this phenomenon?

a.   Supersensitivity.
b.   Idiosyncrasy.
c.   Hypersensitivity.
d.   Tachyphylaxis.
e.   Tolerance.

9 A 66-year-old female is scheduled to undergo a mastectomy with axillary clearance. Her medical history includes hypertension and chronic renal impairment with a glomerular filtration rate of 27ml/minute. Which one of the following analgesics is the most appropriate to use for postoperative pain relief in this patient?

a.   Morphine.
b.   Fentanyl.
c.   Diclofenac.
d.   Tramadol.
e.   Remifentanil.

10 A 59-year-old male is undergoing excision of a noradrenaline-secreting phaeochromocytoma. Intra-operatively he develops severe hypertension. Which one of the following drugs is most suitable in the management of hypertension in this patient?

a.   Glyceryl trinitrate.
b.   Phenoxybenzamine.
c.   Phentolamine.
d.   Labetalol.
e.   Sodium nitroprusside.

11 A 65-year-old man known to have COPD is admitted with severe respiratory distress. What is the flow rate required to deliver 28% oxygen through a venturi mask?

a.   4L/minute.
b.   6L/minute.
c.   8L/minute.
d.   10L/minute.
e.   15L/minute.

12 A 28-year-old primiparous is scheduled for an elective Caesarean section under spinal anaesthesia. Which one of the following is associated with the lowest incidence of postdural puncture headache in this patient?

a.   Performing the procedure in the lateral position.
b.   Using a 22-gauge Sprotte needle instead of a 25-gauge needle.
c.   Using a 22-gauge Quincke needle.
d.   Using a 25-gauge Whitacre needle.
e.   Using a 25-gauge Yale needle.

13 A 27-year-old man is scheduled for removal of a superficial foreign body from his forearm under general anaesthesia. He is ASA 1 and weighs 78kg with a BMI of 28. Which of the following supraglottic airway devices would you choose for securing the airway?

a.   LMA size 6, inflated up to 50ml.
b.   LMA size 5, inflated up to 50ml.
c.   LMA size 5, inflated up to 40ml.
d.   LMA size 4, inflated up to 40ml.
e.   Size 5 i-Gel® supraglottic airway.

14 A patient with cardiogenic shock is having an intra-aortic balloon pump inserted. Which of the following will you rule out before using the pump?

a.   Acute myocardial infarction.
b.   Acute mitral regurgitation.
c.   Aortic regurgitation.
d.   Unstable angina.
e.   Ventricular arrhythmias.

15 As part of awake fibreoptic intubation, you have injected 2ml of 2% lidocaine just below the cornu of the hyoid bone, through the thyrohyoid ligament. Which of the following intrinsic muscles of the larynx is likely to be paralysed?

a.   Transverse arytenoid.
b.   Posterior cricoarytenoid.
c.   Cricothyroid.
d.   Thyroarytenoid.
e.   Aryepiglottics.

16 A 40-year-old male has been asked to perform a Valsalva manoeuvre. Which one of these physiological changes is unlikely to happen during the manoeuvre?

a.   Increased pressure in the intrathoracic arteries.
b.   Pooling of blood in the pulmonary vessels.
c.   Lowering of the blood pressure.
d.   An increase in the interatrial differential pressure.
e.   Rise in heart rate.

17 A 45-year-old man with severe carbon monoxide poisoning is receiving hyperbaric oxygen therapy in a tertiary intensive care unit. Which one of the following physiologic changes is most likely to occur?

a. Reduction in systemic vascular resistance.
b. Reduction in pulmonary vascular resistance.
c. Increased oxygen flux due to a significant increase in oxygen saturation.
d. Unchanged mixed venous oxygen saturation.
e. Increased endothelial neutrophil adhesion.

18 In an adult, about 180L of water is filtered in a day, but in the presence of normal levels of functioning anti-diuretic hormone (ADH) about 99% of the filtered water is reabsorbed. In which one of the following anatomical locations of the kidney is the greatest fraction of filtered water reabsorbed?

a. Proximal convoluted tubule.
b. Ascending loop of Henle.
c. Distal tubule.
d. Cortical collecting duct.
e. Medullary collecting duct.

19 Which of the following statements best describes the functional residual capacity?

a. Sum of expiratory reserve volume and residual volume.
b. Difference between inspiratory capacity and tidal volume.
c. Sum of expiratory reserve volume and tidal volume.
d. Sum of residual volume and tidal volume.
e. Sum of inspiratory reserve volume and tidal volume.

20 Buffers are important in maintaining the acid-base balance in the body. Which one of the following is the most important buffer in interstitial fluid?

a.   Phosphate buffers.
b.   Carbonic acid buffers.
c.   Compounds containing histidine.
d.   Haemoglobin.
e.   Plasma proteins.

21 A 42-year-old female is admitted to the intensive care unit with subarachnoid haemorrhage. Which one of the following drugs would be most effective in the prevention and treatment of ischaemic neurological deficits in this patient?

a.   Nifedipine.
b.   Amlodipine.
c.   Nicorandil.
d.   Nicardipine.
e.   Nimodipine.

22 Drug A has a clearance of 200ml/minute, a duration of action of 500 minutes and is effective at a plasma concentration of 0.02mg/ml. Its bioavailability is 100%. From the above data, which one of the following most likely indicates the required dose in milligrams for oral administration for drug A in an adult?

a.   2000mg.
b.   1000mg.
c.   1500mg.
d.   400mg.
e.   500mg.

23 A 69-year-old male who is a poorly controlled asthmatic falls off a balcony and sustains pelvic trauma. His blood pressure is 60/40mmHg and heart rate is 122/minute. There is no neurological injury and the CT scan of his head is normal. He is scheduled for internal fixation of his pelvis. The most appropriate induction agent would be:

a.   Etomidate.
b.   Thiopentone.
c.   Propofol.
d.   Ketamine.
e.   Inhalational induction with sevoflurane.

24 Which of the following non-steroidal anti-inflammatory drugs (NSAIDs) has the highest risk of a serious gastrointestinal side effect?

a.   Ibuprofen.
b.   Ketorolac.
c.   Diclofenac.
d.   Indomethacin.
e.   Celecoxib.

25 A 56-year-old farmer is admitted to the emergency department with frothy secretions in his mouth, breathlessness, urinary incontinence and sweating. On examination his heart rate is 56 per minute, blood pressure is 110/60mm Hg and pupils are constricted. Which one of the following drugs is the treatment of choice?

a.   Physostigmine.
b.   Atropine.
c.   Naloxone.
d.   Midazolam.
e.   Edrophonium.

26 A pH of 7 = 100nmol/L of H⁺ ions. Which of the following concentrations of hydrogen ions is equivalent to a pH of 9?

a.   1nmol/L.
b.   10nmol/L.
c.   90nmol/L.
d.   100nmol/L.
e.   1000nmol/L.

27 You are anaesthetising a patient at 3 atmospheres. If the flow rate on the anaesthetic machine is 2L/minute, which one of the following indicates the actual delivered flow rate?

a.   2L/minute.
b.   Greater than 2L/minute.
c.   Less than 2L/minute.
d.   4L/minute.
e.   3L/minute.

28 Humidifying inspired gases can be achieved using nebulisers and humidifiers. The droplet size is important when selecting a nebuliser as droplets of 1μm in size are ideal as they reach the alveoli. Which of the following methods is the most efficient in producing droplets of 1μm?

a.   Spinning disc nebuliser.
b.   Heat and moisture exchanger.
c.   Heated water bath.
d.   Ultrasonic nebuliser.
e.   Heated Bernoulli nebuliser.

29 During low-flow anaesthesia, the inspired oxygen concentration in fresh gas flow can be further diluted. Which of the following is most useful in preventing the delivery of hypoxic gas mixtures during low-flow anaesthesia using a fresh gas flow of 0.3L/minute?

a. Mechanical link 25 system.
b. Pneupac ratio system.
c. Penlon electronic system.
d. The Ritchie whistle.
e. Breath-to-breath oxygen monitoring close to the endotracheal tube.

30 Regular maintenance of electrodes in blood gas analyzers is essential. In the CO_2 electrode, which of the following components most needs to be replaced at regular intervals?

a. The membrane covering the electrode.
b. The electrode itself.
c. The electrolyte solution.
d. The pump tubings.
e. The rinsing fluid.

Set 3 answers

1   Answer: C. 26mmol/L.

The anion gap is calculated using the following formula:

$$\text{Anion gap} = Na^+ + [K^+] - HCO_3^- + Cl^-$$
$$= (136 + 4) - (12 + 102) = 26\text{mmol/L}$$

Causes for a low anion gap include laboratory error and hypoalbuminaemia. A low anion gap can also occur in the presence of a paraproteinaemia or intoxication with lithium, bromide, or iodide. A high anion gap commonly indicates metabolic acidosis but can also reflect laboratory error, metabolic alkalosis, hyperphosphataemia, or paraproteinaemia. A normal anion gap is 8-12mmol/L if K^+ is not taken into consideration and 10-18mmol/L if K^+ is taken into consideration.

Metabolic acidosis can be divided into high anion and normal anion gap types which can be present alone or concurrently. This lady has diabetic ketoacidosis, which is a high anion gap metabolic acidosis. A high anion gap acidosis is generally due to the overproduction of organic acids or due to a proportionate reduction in the excretion of anions. In many cases, the identity of anions that contribute to the elevated anion gap can be determined. This is particularly true when the serum anion gap is >30mmol/L, in which case the most common anions found are lactate (lactic acidosis) and β-hydroxybutyrate and acetoacetate (ketoacidosis). However, a small increase in the serum anion gap (anion gap of 24mmol/L or less) can be present without an identifiable, accumulating acid in >30% of cases.

Further reading
1. Kaye AD, Riopelle JM. Intravascular fluid and electrolyte physiology. In: *Miller's anesthesia*, Volume 2, 7th ed. Miller RD, Ed. Philadelphia, USA: Churchill Livingstone, 2010; Chapter 54: 1721-2.

2   Answer: B. High pulmonary artery pressure.

Following birth, pulmonary artery pressures reduce to normal levels within the first 24 hours (at sea level). In babies born at high altitude the pulmonary artery pressures remain elevated for much longer (weeks to months). Pulmonary vasoconstriction would be a response to a hypoxic environment. Variation in heart rate would be minimal. Right atrial pressures would remain higher for a few days to weeks. There would not be any changes in stroke volume. In infants born at high altitude, the transition to adult circulation occurs more slowly. There is an increased frequency of patent foramen ovale and patent ductus arteriosus. Acute hypoxia after birth in preterm infants paradoxically produces hypoventilation, periodic breathing and apnoea.

Further reading
1. Niermeyer S. Cardiopulmoary transition in the high altitude infant. *High Alt Med Biol* 2003; 4: 225-39.
2. Moon RE, Camporesi EM. Clinical care in extreme environments: at high and low pressure and in space. In: *Miller's anesthesia*, Volume 2, 7th ed. Miller RD. Philadelphia, USA: Churchill Livingstone, 2010; Chapter 80: 2503-4.

3   Answer: B. 350ml.

Maximum allowable blood loss (MABL) can be calculated as:

$$MABL = \frac{EBV \times (\text{starting haematocrit - target haematocrit})}{\text{Starting haematocrit}}$$

$$= \frac{(20 \times 70) \times (40 - 30)}{40}$$

$$= 350$$

82

Maximum allowable blood loss (MABL) takes into consideration the patient's age, haematocrit and weight. In general, blood volume is approximately 100 to 120ml/kg for a preterm infant, 90ml/kg for a full-term infant, 80ml/kg for a child 3 to 12 months old, and 70ml/kg for a child older than 1 year. These are merely estimates of blood volume. The individual child's blood volume is calculated by simple proportion by multiplying the child's weight by the estimated blood volume (EBV) per kilogram. MABL would be replaced with 3ml of lactated Ringer's solution per ml of blood loss; that is, 3ml of lactated Ringer's solution times the 350ml of blood loss equals approximately 1050ml of lactated Ringer's solution. If blood loss is less than or equal to MABL and no further significant blood loss occurs or is anticipated in the postoperative period, there is no need for transfusion of red blood cells (RBCs). However, if significant postoperative bleeding occurs or is anticipated, it is very important to discuss the potential transfusion needs with the surgeon. If the child has reached the MABL and significantly more blood loss is expected during surgery, the child should receive RBCs in sufficient quantity to maintain the haematocrit in the 20% to 25% range. Haematocrit values in the low 20% range are generally well tolerated by most children, the exception being preterm infants, term newborns, and children with cyanotic congenital heart disease or those with respiratory failure in need of a high oxygen-carrying capacity.

Further reading
1. Cote CJ. Paediatric anesthesia. In: *Miller's anesthesia*, Volume 2, 7th ed. Miller RD. Philadelphia, USA: Churchill Livingstone, 2010; Chapter 82: 2581-4.

4 Answer: C. Increased free fatty acids.

During the 24 to 48 hours after cessation of nutrient intake, glycogen stores are broken down (glycogenolysis) to maintain basal plasma glucose levels. This glucose is vital for the brain, red blood cells, skin and renal medulla, which have obligatory glucose requirements. Glycogenolysis is mediated by an increased glucagon/insulin ratio (increased glucagon and decreased insulin), which also promotes endogenous glucose production (gluconeogenesis). In addition to the increases in glucagon and decreases in insulin, hypoglycaemia is avoided by small increases in catecholamine and cortisol secretion. As starvation continues, skeletal and smooth muscle tissues undergo proteolysis (increased protein breakdown) to amino acids, which are used as substrates for gluconeogenesis. This muscle breakdown results in a negative nitrogen balance. During this time the majority of ATP is produced from fatty acids released by lipolysis. The increase in catecholamine-induced β-adrenergic stimulation accelerates lipolysis so that triglycerides stored in adipose tissue are broken down to free fatty acids (FFA) and glycerol. Some of the FFA undergo hepatic conversion to ketones (β-hydroxybutyrate and acetoacetate), which are then utilised as an energy source. Ketone levels are raised as a result of increasing fat metabolism. Magnesium levels are not usually affected in acute starvation, though chronic starvation and dieting can lower the levels significantly.

Further reading
1. Hall JE. Dietary balances; Regulation of feeding; Obesity and starvation; Vitamins and Minerals. In: *Guyton and Hall textbook of medical physiology*, 12th ed. Philadelphia, USA: Elsevier Saunders, 2011; Unit XIII, Chapter 71: 843-52.
2. Weissman C. Nutrition and metabolic control. In: *Miller's anesthesia*, Volume 2, 7th ed. Miller RD. Philadelphia, USA: Churchill Livingstone, 2010; Chapter 95: 2923-44.

5   Answer: B. Reduced FEV1.

In smokers, blood concentration of carbon monoxide is increased to as much as 10%. Carbon monoxide has a higher affinity to bind to haemoglobin than oxygen (250 times higher), thus making less haemoglobin available for oxygen binding. This shifts the oxygen dissociation curve to the left, which reduces the release of oxygen to the tissues. The forced expiratory volume at 1 second (FEV1) starts to decline at the rate of 60ml per year as compared to 20ml per year in non-smokers. Chronic smoking causes a reduction in FEV1 and the FEV1/FVC ratio.

Upper and lower airway reactivity is increased in smokers. This coupled with impaired mucociliary transport increases the risk of peri-operative laryngospasm, bronchospasm and atelectasis in smokers. Forced vital capacity is usually reduced in smokers.

Further reading
1. Moppett I, Curran J. Smoking and the surgical patient. *British Journal of Anaestheisa CEACCP* 2001; 1: 122-4.

6   Answer: D. Synergism.

Drug interactions are described by various terminologies. These include summation, antagonism, potentiation, and synergism. These terms are defined as follows.

◆ Summation - this indicates the additive effects of two or more similarly acting drugs, e.g. combined effect of nitrous oxide and sevoflurane.
◆ Antagonism - there are different types of antagonistic drug interactions. These can be chemical antagonism (protamine and heparin), pharmacokinetic antagonism (enzyme inhibition) or receptor antagonism. Receptor antagonism may further be classified as reversible (e.g. morphine and naloxone) or irreversible (e.g. phenoxybenzamine and noradrenaline).
◆ Potentiation - in this phenomenon, the effects of one drug are enhanced by another drug by pharmacokinetic interaction (e.g. enzyme inhibition or displacement from protein binding sites). The two drugs involved generally have different pharmacodynamic activity (digoxin and thiazide diuretic).
◆ Synergism or supra-additive effect - two drugs with similar pharmacological properties and closely related sites of action produce an effect in combination, which is greater than the additive effect.

Further reading
1. Calvey TN, Williams NE. Drug interaction. In: *Principles and practice of pharmacology for anaesthetists*, 4th ed. Oxford, UK: Blackwell Science, 2001: 64-5.

7 Answer: B. Morphine.

Selegiline is a selective inhibitor of type B monoamine oxidase. Monoamine oxidase (MAO) inhibitors are also used as antidepressant drugs. They interfere with metabolism of monoamines (dopamine, tyramine) and can affect biotransformation of drugs such as pethidine and dextromethorphan. The interaction with opioid analgesics may be excitatory (agitation, hypertension, pyrexia, tachyarrhythmia, convulsions) or inhibitory (hypotension, hypoventilation, coma).

These drugs act indirectly via catecholamine release (ephedrine, metaraminol), and oral ingestion of tyramine-rich food (cheese, red wine) can also interact with MAO inhibitors. Doxapram is also considered unsafe to use in a patient on MAO inhibitors.

Further reading
1. Calvey TN, Williams NE. Drug interaction. In: *Principles and practice of pharmacology for anaesthetists*, 4th ed. Oxford, UK: Blackwell Science, 2001: 79-80.
2. Peck T, Wong A, Norman E. Anaesthetic implications of psychoactive drugs. *British Journal of Anaesthesia CEACCP* 2010; 10: 177-81.

8 Answer: B. Idiosyncrasy.

The response to a particular drug varies and this could be due to idiosyncracy, supersensitivity, tachyphylaxis, tolerance or hypersensitivity. Idiosyncracy is a genetically determined abnormal reaction (extreme sensitivity or marked insensitivity) to a drug, e.g. malignant hyperpyrexia, acute hepatic porphyria.

In acute hepatic porphyria, enzyme-inducing drugs (barbiturates, alcohol, phenytoin, oral contraceptives) increase activity of δ-aminolevulinic acid (ALA) synthetase leading to an increased production of porphyrins. This leads to widespread demyelination of peripheral and central pathways causing sensory changes and motor paralysis.

Supersensitivity can occur due to up-regulation of receptors (e.g. following denervation) and this leads to an exaggerated response to a particular drug (significant hyperkalaemia after suxamethonium administration to patients with spinal cord injury or severe burn).

Tachyphylaxis is a rapid decrease in response to identical doses of an agonist within a short period of time.

Tolerance is a gradual decrease in the activity of drugs, which usually occurs over a period of days or weeks (e.g. decreasing effect of opioid after long-term use due to down-regulation of receptors).

Hypersensitivity is an immunologically-mediated abnormal reaction to a drug and usually involves the formation of antibodies.

Further reading
1. Calvey TN, Williams NE. Variability in drug response. In: *Principles and practice of pharmacology for anaesthetists*, 4th ed. Oxford, UK: Blackwell Science, 2001: 93-5.

9   Answer: B. Fentanyl.

This patient has impaired renal function with a severe reduction in glomerular filtration rate. Non-steroidal anti-inflammatory drugs would further deteriorate renal function due to their effect on renal blood flow and for this reason diclofenac should be avoided in this patient. Both morphine and tramadol have active metabolites, which are excreted via the kidney. The active metabolites of these drugs may accumulate in this patient causing toxicity. Fentanyl is predominantly metabolized in the liver and about 70% of administered dose is excreted in the urine as inactive metabolites. Although remifentanil does not depend on the kidney for excretion, its use in the management of postoperative pain is limited.

Further reading
1. Calvey TN, Williams NE. Analgesic drugs. In: *Principles and practice of pharmacology for anaesthetists*, 4th ed. Oxford, UK: Blackwell Science, 2001: 208-9.

10 Answer: C. Phentolamine.

Severe hypertension, intra-operatively, in a patient undergoing phaeochromocytoma excision surgery is usually caused by a release of catecholamines on handling of the tumour. If it is a noradrenaline-secreting tumour, the hypertension is most appropriately managed by using intravenous phentolamine. Phentolamine has a shorter duration of action than phenoxybenzamine.

Phenoxybenzamine is commonly used pre-operatively to stabilise hypertension in patients awaiting phaeochromocytoma excision surgery.

Further reading
1. Calvey TN, Williams NE. The autonomic nervous system. In: *Principles and practice of pharmacology for anaesthetists*, 4th ed. Oxford, UK: Blackwell Science, 2001: 266-7.

11 Answer: A. 4L/minute.

The FiO_2 delivered by venturi mask depends on the oxygen flow rate and the amount of air entrained. The amount of air entrained depends on the venturi mask adaptors. There are slits in the venturi mask adaptors, which become smaller or larger depending on whether a high or lower FIO_2 is required. These slits are designed to entrain air from the environment. Therefore, the set oxygen flow and the entrained air together meet the inspiratory flow requirement of the patient. The average FiO_2 (fraction of inspired oxygen) delivered through venturi masks can be up to 5% above the expected value.

Venturi masks provide a higher gas flow than the peak inspiratory flow rate irrespective of the patient's respiratory pattern. The FiO_2 delivered depends on the combination of venturi mask adaptor and the oxygen flow rate. Therefore, just increasing the oxygen flow rate but keeping the adaptor constant does not increase the FiO_2 delivered.

Venturi adaptors and oxygen flow rates are shown in Table 1.

FiO$_2$	Colour coding	Oxygen flow L/min
0.24	Blue	2
0.28	White	4
0.31	Brown	6
0.35	Yellow	8
0.40	Red	10
0.60	Green	15

Table 1. Venturi adaptors and oxygen flow rates.

Further reading
1. Al-Shaikh B, Stacey S, Eds. Fixed performance devices. In: *Essentials of anaesthetic equipment*, 3rd ed. London, UK: Churchill Livingstone, Elsevier, 2007; Chapter 6: 89-91.

12 Answer: D. Using a 25-gauge Whitacre needle.

The incidence of postdural puncture headache (PDPH) increases with the size of the needle (a 22G needle is bigger than a 25G) and decreases with increasing age of the patient. The risk of dural headache is higher in pregnancy and labour. Cutting needles (Quincke, Yale) are likely to increase the risk compared to atraumatic needles (Sprotte, Whitacre). Meta-analyses conclude that a non-cutting needle should be used for patients at high risk of PDPH, and the smallest gauge needle available should be used for all patients. The position of the patient whilst performing the procedure does not affect the incidence of PDPH.

Further reading
1. Al-Shaikh B, Stacey S, Eds. Pain management and regional anaesthesia. In: *Essentials of anaesthetic equipment*, 3rd ed. London, UK: Churchill Livingstone, Elsevier, 2007; Chapter 12: 186-7.

2. Lambert DH, Hurley RJ, Hertwig L, Datta S. Role of needle gauge and tip configuration in the production of lumbar puncture headache. *Regional Anesthesia* 1997; 22: 66-72.

13 Answer: C. LMA size 5, inflated up to 40ml.

A size 5 LMA is used for adults weighing 70 to 100kg. The manufacturers state that the maximum recommended cuff volume should never be exceeded and inflation pressure should be <60cm H_2O. Nitrous oxide diffuses into cuffs and will increase pressures. In several studies, the incidence of sore throat was significantly reduced if 'just-seal' or half of the maximum recommended volume was used. A hyperinflated cuff may be displaced from the pharynx with loss of seal and be too rigid to adapt to the contours of the pharynx. Hyperinflated cuffs have been implicated in direct compression of pharyngeal structures and paralysis of recurrent laryngeal and hypoglossal nerves in children. Hence, an optimally sized LMA must be selected rather than overinflating a small LMA. A size 5 i-Gel® supraglottic airway is suitable for patients weighing greater than 90kg.

Further reading
1. Al-Shaikh B, Stacey S, Eds. Tracheal and tracheostomy tubes and airways. In: *Essentials of anaesthetic equipment*, 3rd ed, London, UK: Churchill Livingstone, Elsevier, 2007; Chapter 5: 80.
2. Patel B, Bingham R. Laryngeal mask airway and other supraglottic airway devices in paediatric practice. *British Journal of Anaesthesia CEACCP* 2009; 9: 6-9.
3. Cook T, Howes B. Supraglottic airway devices: recent advances. *British Journal of Anaesthesia CEACCP* 2011; 11: 56-61.

14 Answer: C. Aortic regurgitation.

An intra-aortic balloon pump (IABP) is a circulatory assist device in critically ill patients with cardiac disease. The basic principle is counter pulsation. The balloon is inflated in diastole and deflated in early systole. Balloon inflation in diastole causes volume displacement of blood within the aorta, both proximally and distally. This leads to a potential increase in coronary blood flow and systemic perfusion by augmentation of the intrinsic Windkessel effect, whereby potential energy stored in the aortic root during systole is converted to kinetic energy with the elastic recoil of the aortic root.

Indications for IABP include the following:

- Acute myocardial infarction.
- Cardiogenic shock.
- Acute mitral regurgitation and ventricular septal defect.
- Catheterisation and angioplasty.
- Refractory unstable angina.
- Refractory ventricular arrhythmias.
- Refractory left ventricular failure.
- Sepsis.

Absolute contra-indications for IABP are:

- Aortic regurgitation.
- Aortic dissection.
- Aortic stents.
- Chronic end-stage heart disease with no anticipation of recovery.

Further reading
1. Krishna M, Zacharowski M. Principles of intra-aortic balloon pump counterpulsation. *British Journal of Anaesthesia CEACCP* 2009; 9: 24-8.

15 Answer: C. Cricothyroid.

The mucosa of the larynx above the level of the vocal cords is anaesthetised by blocking the superior laryngeal nerve (SLN). SLN block can be performed externally by injecting local anaesthetic just caudal to the greater cornu of the hyoid bone. The SLN divides into two branches, internal and external. The internal laryngeal nerve pierces the thyrohyoid membrane and provides sensory innervation to the mucosa above the level of the vocal cords. The external laryngeal nerve provides motor innervation to one intrinsic muscle of the larynx (cricothyroid). With the exception of cricothyroid, all the other intrinsic muscles of the larynx are innervated by the recurrent laryngeal nerve.

Further reading

1. The larynx. In: *Anatomy for anaesthetists*, 8th ed. Ellis H, Feldman S, Harrop-Griffiths W, Eds. Oxford, UK: Blackwell Publishing Ltd, 2004; part 1: 26-37.

16 Answer: D. An increase in the interatrial differential pressure.

The Valsalva manoeuvre refers to the forced expiration against a closed glottis after a full inspiration. The normal physiological response consists of four phases:

- ◆ Phase I - an increase in the intrathoracic pressures expels the blood from the thoracic blood vessels. This causes a rise in blood pressure.
- ◆ Phase II - the increase in intrathoracic pressure causes a drop in the venous return, lowering the preload and BP. The baroreceptor reflex is then activated, which causes vasoconstriction and tachycardia.
- ◆ Phase III - when pressure is released, the intrathoracic pressure suddenly decreases resulting in pooling of blood in the pulmonary vessels, which causes a further drop in BP.
- ◆ Phase IV - with venous return restored there is an overshoot as compensatory mechanisms continue to operate. The increased BP causes a baroreceptor-mediated bradycardia.

Further reading

1. Yentis SM, Hirsch NP, Smith GB, Eds. Valsalva manoeuvre. In: *Anaesthesia and intensive care. A-Z - An encyclopedia of principles and practice*, 3rd ed. Philadelphia, USA: Elsevier, 2005: 529-30.

17 Answer: B. Reduction in pulmonary vascular resistance.

Breathing oxygen at increased ambient pressure will lead to an elevation of alveolar O_2 tension (PAO_2). Whilst breathing oxygen at 1 atmosphere absolute (ATA) pressure, the fraction of O_2 in arterial blood that is carried in the dissolved form is minimal. At a pressure of 2 to 3 ATA, PaO_2 increases and the amount of oxygen dissolved in plasma increases significantly. Increased PaO_2 results in increased oxygen content and vasoconstriction in systemic vessels.

Hyperbaric oxygen (HBO) causes an increase in systemic vascular resistance by inactivation of nitric oxide due to increased production of superoxide and possibly decreased release of nitric oxide from circulating S-nitrosohaemoglobin. Hypoxia causes pulmonary vasoconstriction, whereas oxygen at increased ambient pressure has the opposite effect and reduces pulmonary arterial pressures. An increase in mixed venous partial pressure of oxygen and oxygen saturation is noted during hyperbaric oxygen therapy.

Increased PaO_2 inhibits endothelial neutrophil adhesion in injured tissue. It also promotes enhanced macrophage interleukin-10 expression and other anti-inflammatory effects.

Further reading
1. Moon RE, Camporesi EM. Clinical care in extreme environments: at high and low pressure and in space. In: *Miller's anesthesia*, Volume 2, 7th ed. Miller RD, Ed. Philadelphia, USA: Churchill Livingstone, 2010; Chapter 80: 2485-99.

18 Answer: A. Proximal convoluted tubule.

Normally, 180L of water is filtered though the glomeruli in a 24-hour period. About 60-70% of this is reabsorbed in the proximal convoluted tubule (PCT). Therefore, the greatest fraction of water is reabsorbed in the PCT irrespective of anti-diuretic hormone (ADH) secretion. ADH increases permeability of the collecting ducts to water, therefore increasing water reabsorption in the collecting ducts. But ADH is responsible for only 10% of the total water absorption by the kidney.

Further reading
1. Ganong WF, Ed. Water excretion. In: *Review of medical physiology,* 22nd ed. New York, USA: McGraw-Hill, 2005; Section 8, Chapter 38: 713-20.

19 Answer: A. Sum of expiratory reserve volume and residual volume.

The functional residual capacity (FRC) is the volume of gas remaining in the lung at the end of a normal expiration. It is the sum of expiratory reserve volume and residual volume. At the point of FRC the ability of the thoracic cage to expand and the elastic recoil of the lung to collapse cancel each other and, hence, FRC represents a state of equilibrium.

The gas in the FRC after a normal expiration acts as a reserve in the lung so that gas exchange continues to take place without interruption. Pre-oxygenation at induction of anaesthesia denitrogenates the FRC volume of air in the lungs. This will be an additional oxygen reserve, particularly useful, if the patient has to be apnoeic for some time. Therefore, any factor that decreases the FRC can increase the rate of desaturation at induction.

The FRC is increased in chronic obstructive airway diseases and during positive intrathoracic pressure.

Inspiratory capacity is the sum of inspiratory reserve volume and tidal volume. Therefore, the difference between inspiratory capacity and tidal volume is the inspiratory reserve volume. Residual volume is the volume of air remaining in the lungs after full expiration.

Further reading
1. Lumb AB, Ed. Lung volumes. In: *Nunn's applied respiratory physiology*, 7th ed. London, UK: Churchill Livingstone, Elsevier, 2010; Chapter 3: 36-41.

20 Answer: B. Carbonic acid buffers.

There are various buffers in different compartments of the body. In blood the most important buffers are carbonic anhydrase, plasma proteins and haemoglobin. In interstitial fluid, the main buffer is carbonic acid. The amount of phosphate present in the plasma is too low to be an effective buffer. Intracellularly, phosphate and protein buffers play an important role. Haemoglobin in the blood has six times the buffering capacity of proteins due to the large amount of haemoglobin present in blood.

The amount of CO_2 dissolved in the blood is controlled by respiration, and the plasma concentration of HCO_3^- is controlled by the renal system. Therefore, carbonic acid/bicarbonate is the most effective buffering system.

Further reading
1. Ganong WF, Ed. Regulation of extracellular fluid composition and volume. In: *Review of medical physiology*, 22nd ed. New York, USA: McGraw-Hill, 2005; Section 8, Chapter 39: 729- 38.

21 Answer: E. Nimodipine.

Nimodipine is a calcium channel blocker, which acts preferentially on cerebral arterioles. It should be administered within 4 days of a subarachnoid hemorrhage and is continued for 3 weeks.

The side effects of nimodipine include hypotension, flushing, sweating, oedema, nausea and other gastrointestinal problems. It is contraindicated in unstable angina and within a month of myocardial infarction.

Nifedipine, nicardipine and amlodipine are also calcium channel blockers but they are not used for the prevention of vasospasm in subarachnoid haemorrhage. Nicorandil is a potassium channel activator used in the treatment of angina.

Further reading
1. Calvey TN, Williams NE. Calcium channel blockers. In: *Principles and practice of pharmacology for anaesthetists*, 4th ed. Oxford, UK: Blackwell Science, 2001; Chapter 14: 301-2.

22   Answer: A. 2000mg.

The required oral dose of a given drug can be calculated by the following equation:

$$\text{The required dose (mg)} =$$

$$\frac{Cp \times I \times CL}{F} = 0.02 \times 500 \times 200/1 = 0.02 \times 100,000$$

$$= 2000$$

Where Cp = the concentration required to produce a given effect (mg/ml); I = the dosage interval in minutes; CL = the clearance of a drug (ml/min); F = the fraction of the dose that enters the systemic circulation (bioavailability in fraction).

Further reading
1. Calvey TN, Williams NE. Pharmacokinetics. In: *Principles and practice of pharmacology for anaesthetists*, 4th ed. Oxford, UK: Blackwell Science, 2001; Chapter 2: 24-5.

23   Answer: D. Ketamine.

The patient has fallen off a balcony and has probably suffered a major haemorrhage due to major pelvic trauma. He is in shock and is wheezy. Propofol and thiopentone should not be used here as they can worsen his hypotension and may lead to cardiac arrest at induction. Whilst etomidate is more cardiostable, ketamine is a better choice as it would help maintain his blood pressure and is also a bronchodilator. Inhalational induction is not appropriate for this situation.

Further reading
1. Pai A, Heining M. Ketamine. *British Journal of Anaesthesia CEACCP* 2007; 7: 59-63
2. Bell RF, Dhai JB, Moore RA, Kalso E. Peri-operative ketamine for acute postoperative pain, a quantitative and qualitative review (Cochrane review). *Acta Anaesthesiol Scand* 2005; 49: 1405-28.

24 Answer: B. Ketorolac.

Non-selective NSAIDs are associated with a higher risk of developing serious gastrointestinal events than selective NSAIDs (coxibs). Of the non-selective NSAIDs, azapropazone is associated with the highest risk, with piroxicam, ketorolac, ketoprofen the next highest risk. NSAIDs that have intermediate risks of causing serious gastrointestinal events include diclofenac, indomethacin and naproxen. The lowest risk is associated with ibuprofen although at high doses ibuprofen is associated with an intermediate risk.

Further reading
1. Reducing NSAID-induced gastro-intestinal complications. *Drug and Therapeutic Bulletin* 2011; 49: 18-21.

25 Answer: B. Atropine.

The most likely diagnosis is an overdose of organophosphate compound, which has cholinergic properties. Organophosphates are highly lipid-soluble agents and are well absorbed from the skin, oral mucous membrane, conjunctiva and gastrointestinal tract. They inactivate the acetylcholinesterases resulting in accumulation of acetylcholine.

The clinical features are related to increased parasympathetic activity, due to accumulation of acetylcholine at both muscarinic and nicotinic sites. These include increased secretions (salivation, lacrimation and sweating), bronchospasm, bradycardia, increased gastrointestinal motility and constricted pupils due to accumulation of acetylcholine at muscarinic sites. Increased acetylcholine at the neuromuscular junction causes muscle fasciculations and flaccid paralysis.

The management involves an airway, breathing and circulation approach. The general measures include skin decontamination, gastric lavage and activated charcoal.

Atropine antagonizes the muscarinic effects of organophosphate on the central nervous system, cardiovascular system and gastrointestinal tract.

The other drug used in the treatment of organophosphate poisoning is pralidoxime (PAM), which re-activates the phosphorylated acetylcholinesterase.

Physostigmine is an anticholinesterase that has a quaternary amine structure and crosses the blood brain barrier. It increases the acetylcholine levels and worsens the clinical features of organophosphate poisoning.

Naloxone is an opioid antagonist used for reversing the effects of opioids. Midazolam can be used as a sedative agent to facilitate ventilatory support. Edrophonium is an anticholinesterase but with a short duration of action as compared with neostigmine and physostigmine.

Further reading

1. Peck TE, Hill SA, Williams M, Eds. Anticholinesterases. In: *Pharmacology for anaesthesia and intensive care*, 3rd ed. Cambridge, UK: Cambridge University Press, 2008; Chapter 11: 192- 6.
2. Kamanyire R, Karalliedde L. Organophosphate toxicity and occupational exposure. *Occupational Medicine* 2004; 54: 69-75.

26   Answer: A. 1nmol/L.

pH is a measure of hydrogen ion activity in a liquid. The pH is defined as the negative logarithm to the base of 10 of [H^+]. A decrease of one pH unit is equivalent to a 10-fold increase of [H^+]:

- pH of 9 = 1nmol/l [H^+] or 10^{-9} mol/L.
- pH of 8 = 10nmol/l [H^+] or 10^{-8} mol/L.
- pH of 7 = 100nmol/l [H^+] or 10^{-7} mol/L.
- pH of 7.4 = 40nmol/l [H^+] or $10^{-7.4}$ mol/L.

The relationship between [H^+] and pH is approximately linear over the middle of the clinical range, the pH decreasing by approximately 0.1 for each 10nmol/L increase in [H^+]. Thus, 50nmol/L corresponds to a pH of 7.3.

Further reading
1. Davis PD, Kenny GNC. Hydrogen ion and carbon dioxide measurement. In: *Basic physics and measurement in anaesthesia*, 5th ed. London, UK: Butterworth-Heinemann, 2003; Chapter 19: 211.

27 Answer: C. Less than 2L/minute.

As atmospheric pressure is increased, the density of gases increases. Therefore, a given amount of gas occupies a lesser volume than at sea level. Less flow is required to maintain the bobbin at a certain height, as it is the number of gas molecules, which support the bobbin. Therefore, the flow meter will over-read at higher atmospheric pressure.

Further reading:
1. Carter JA. Provision of anaesthesia in difficult situations and the developing world. In: *Ward's anaesthetic equipment*, 5th ed. Davey AJ, Diba A, Eds. Philadelphia, USA, Elsevier Saunders, 2005; Chapter 29: 485-98.

28 Answer: D: Ultrasonic nebuliser.

A spinning disc nebuliser is a motor-driven spinning disc which throws out water droplets by centrifugal force.

The heat and moisture exchanger (HME) retains moisture and heat from the expired gas and returns this to the inspired gas during the next inspiration. An inspired gas humidity of $25g/m^3$ can be achieved by HMEs. However, their efficiency is reduced over time by secretions.

In heated water bath humidifiers, water is heated to a desired temperature. The dry gas enters the container and becomes saturated with water vapour. This is then delivered to the breathing system.

In ultrasonic nebulisers, a transducer head vibrates at a frequency of around 3Hz, producing droplets of less than 1 to 2μm in size. Droplets greater than 5μm are deposited in the upper airway. Droplets of 2-6μm are deposited in the tracheobronchial airways and droplets of 1μm size reach the alveoli.

Further reading

1. Wilkes AR. Humidification: its importance and delivery. *British Journal of Anaesthesia CEPD Review* 2001; 1: 40-3.
2. Davis PD, Kenny GNC. Humidification. In: *Basic physics and measurement in anaesthesia*, 5th ed. London, UK: Butterworth-Heinemann, 2003: 127-36.

29 Answer: E. Breath-to-breath oxygen monitoring close to the endotracheal tube.

When oxygen and nitrous oxide are used, it is possible to deliver a hypoxic gas mixture, if inspired oxygen concentration is not constantly monitored. A mechanical link 25 system uses a chain to link flow control valves for oxygen and nitrous oxide. This system may fail to account for other gases, such as air, reducing the oxygen concentration to less than 25%.

A Pneupac ratio system uses a ratio mixer valve. Oxygen supplied to this valve exerts a pressure on one side of the diaphragm, which is opposed by the pressure of nitrous oxide on the opposite side. The diaphragm construction ensures an increase in oxygen flow rate by a ratio of 25% of any increase in the nitrous oxide flow rate.

Electronic devices (e.g. Penlon) use a paramagnetic oxygen analyser to continuously sample the gas mixtures from the flow meters. If the inspired oxygen fraction decreases below 0.25, the nitrous oxide is temporarily cut off, whereas an increase in the inspired oxygen fraction will temporarily restore nitrous oxide flow.

All of the above three systems ensure that a minimum of 25% oxygen is delivered from the common gas outlet. However, during low-flow anaesthesia, other gases and vapours dilute the inspired oxygen concentration in the breathing system. Therefore, a system that ensures 25% oxygen concentration at the common gas outlet is not sufficient in preventing the delivery of a hypoxic mixture to the patient. The inspired oxygen concentration needs to be monitored close to the endotracheal tube to avoid delivering hypoxic gas mixtures.

The Ritchie whistle is powered by an oxygen supply at a pressure of 420kPa. At a pressure below 200kPa it cuts off the supply of anaesthetic gases and allows the patient to inspire room air. The whistle sounds continuously until the pressure has fallen to 40.5kPa.

Further reading
1. Sinclair CM, Thadsad MK, Barker I. Modern anaesthetic machines. *British Journal of Anaesthesia CEACCP* 2006; 6: 75-8.
2. Diba A. The anaesthetic workstation. In: *Ward's anaesthetic equipment*, 5th ed. Davey AJ, Diba A, Eds. Philadelphia, USA: Elsevier Saunders, 2005; Chapter 6: 106-15.

30 Answer: A. The membrane covering the electrode.

In the CO_2 electrode, CO_2 diffuses through the membrane and reacts with water in the electrolyte solution to produce hydrogen ions. The hydrogen ion concentration is measured with a pH-sensitive glass electrode. As with other electrodes, the CO_2 electrode needs regular maintenance. Integrity of the membrane is essential for the accuracy of the electrode. If a hole occurs in the membrane it ceases to be a semi-permeable membrane.

The CO_2 electrode is calibrated using two different gases with known concentrations of CO_2. The electrode itself does not require regular replacement, but other components such as pump tubing, calibrating solution and rinse fluid should be replaced at regular intervals.

In the automated modern blood gas analyser, by selecting the analyser status screen on the display monitor, the time for electrode and membrane replacement can be checked.

Further reading
1. Al-Shaikh B, Stacey S, Eds. Arterial blood gases analyser. In: *Essentials of anaesthetic equipment*, 3rd ed. London, UK: Churchill Livingstone, Elsevier, 2007: 164-7.

Set 4 questions

1   Normally blood takes 0.75s to traverse the pulmonary capillaries at rest. If this time is reduced to 0.2s, which one of the following gases reaches equilibrium between the alveoli and capillary blood?

a.   Oxygen.
b.   Carbon dioxide.
c.   Carbon monoxide.
d.   Nitrous oxide.
e.   Nitrogen.

2   A young male patient has a haemoglobin concentration of 10g/dL and his peripheral oxygen saturation (SpO_2) is 100%. The oxygen carrying capacity of his blood would be:

a.   20.8ml/dL.
b.   11.1ml/dL.
c.   10.4ml/dL.
d.   13.4ml/dL.
e.   16.6ml/dL.

3   After general anaesthesia, the oxygen content of a preterm neonate is likely to fall because of all these reasons except:

a.   Possibility of apnoeic spells.
b.   Low haemoglobin concentration.
c.   Low oxygen reserve.
d.   Increased oxygen consumption.
e.   Respiratory muscle fatigue.

4   A 60-year-old gentleman has presented with chronic severe pain in his right leg which could not be controlled with medication. His chronic pain physician plans a cordotomy. Which one of the following spinal tracts is interrupted during cordotomy?

a.   Left ventral spinothalamic tract.
b.   Left dorsal column.
c.   Right lateral spinothalamic tract.
d.   Right corticospinal tract.
e.   Left lateral spinothalamic tract.

5   Which one of the following plasma proteins has the greatest effect on plasma colloid osmotic pressure?

a.   Albumin.
b. α-1 globulin.
c. α-2 globulin.
d. β globulin.
e.   Gamma globulin.

6   A 60-year-old male patient with shortness of breath is diagnosed with pulmonary fibrosis. His other medical history includes atrial fibrillation, hyperchloesterolaemia and hypertension. Which one of the following medications could be responsible?

a.   Warfarin.
b.   Simvastatin.
c.   Amiodarone.
d.   Atenolol.
e.   Furosemide.

7   Analgesics such as fentanyl can be administered using a transdermal route. Which one of the following properties is most important for transdermal delivery of a drug?

a.   High molecular weight.
b.   Long terminal half-life.
c.   Non-ionised form.
d.   Low potency.
e.   Highly hydrophobic.

8   A 54-year-old male patient is undergoing an emergency laparotomy for a perforated duodenal ulcer. His medical history includes hypertension, depression and hypothyroidism. During the intra-operative period, a 9mg bolus of ephedrine was given to treat an episode of hypotension. Subsequently he developed severe tachycardia and hypertension. Which one of the following medications could have contributed to this?

a.   Doxazocin.
b.   Fosinopril.
c.   Thyroxine.
d.   Phenelzine.
e.   Aspirin.

9   There are a number of drugs that inhibit the various iso-enzymes of the phosphodiesterase (PDE) enzyme. Which of the following PDE inhibitors has an antiplatelet effect?

a.   Milrinone.
b.   Clopidogrel.
c.   Enoximone.
d.   Dipyridamole.
e.   Amrinone.

10 A young female patient that is suspected to have deliberately self-harmed is admitted to the emergency department. She gives a history of severe depression and was found with an empty bottle of aspirin. An arterial blood gas analysis was performed on arrival to the accident and emergency department. Which of the following parameters suggests an aspirin overdose?

a. PaO_2 of 10kPa.
b. $PaCO_2$ of 2.9kPa.
c.   pH of 7.32.
d.   BE of 4mmol/L.
e. K^+ of 5.0mmol/L.

11 Which one of the following most accurately represents the precautions taken to minimise the risk of fire and explosion in the theatre environment?

a.   The relative humidity in theatre should be at least 85%.
b.   Substitution of cotton fabric with nylon.
c.   Use of only CO_2 as insufflation gas during laparoscopic surgery.
d.   Maintaining a 10cm zone of risk around the anaesthetic machine.
e.   Maintaining a maximum number of six air changes per hour.

12 A young male has developed a spontaneous pneumothorax. On arrival to the accident and emergency department a chest drain has been inserted. Which one of the following features of the underwater seal chest drain system is most essential to facilitate safe and effective drainage?

a.   The drain should be at least 100cm below the level of the chest.
b.   The diameter of the drain tube should be as small as possible.
c.   The volume of the drain tube should be more than 50% of the patient's maximal inspiratory volume.
d.   The drain tube should be at least 10cm below the surface of water.
e.   A suction of up to -50cm H_2O should be applied.

13 Which one of the following is the most appropriate technique to effectively disinfect a fibreoptic endoscope?

a. Formaldehyde gas sterilisation.
b. Ethylene oxide sterilisation.
c. Immersion in quaternary ammonium compound solution for 20 minutes.
d. Immersion in 2% glutaraldehyde solution.
e. Steam sterilisation.

14 For spontaneous ventilation, the Mapleson system A (Magill's circuit) is the most efficient system. What is the single most important reason for this?

a. Requires low fresh gas flow.
b. Does not allow wastage of fresh gas flow.
c. Dead space gas is re-used.
d. Fresh gas flow is equal to alveolar ventilation.
e. It is cheap.

15 Medical monitoring equipment is classified according to the means of protection it provides against electric shock. Which of the following statements best describes class 2 equipment?

a. Any conducting part that is accessible to the user is connected to the earth without a fuse in the mains plug.
b. It is double insulated equipment and is connected to the earth with a fuse in the main plug.
c. It is double insulated equipment and the earth wire is not essential.
d. It is internally powered equipment with minimal risk of electric shock.
e. It is double insulated equipment with no risk of microshock.

16 Pre-oxygenation during induction of anaesthesia delays the onset of critical hypoxia during the period of apnoea. Which of the following best describes the mechanism involved in pre-oxygenation?

a.   It replaces nitrogen in the FRC with oxygen.
b.   It increases the concentration of inspired oxygen.
c.   It increases the amount of dissolved oxygen in blood.
d.   It increases the peripheral oxygen saturation.
e.   It decreases the shunt fraction.

17 An obese 80-year-old gentleman presents for a cystoscopy. He is previously fit and well. General anaesthesia is induced and the airway is secured with an LMA. He is breathing 28% oxygen spontaneously. Ten minutes later his oxygen saturation decreases from 99% to 96%. Which of the following statements best describes the reason for this?

a.   Increased sensitivity to hypoxia and hypercarbia in the elderly.
b.   Increased residual volume in the elderly.
c.   Absorption atelectasis.
d.   Reduced FRC due to supine position and general anaesthesia.
e.   The loss of auto-PEEP due to the presence of the LMA.

18 A young female is undergoing reconstructive free flap surgery as part of the removal of a malignant tumour. The surgeon is very concerned about flap survival. Which of the following describes the best way to promote blood flow and tissue perfusion in the free flap?

a.   Maintaining a MAP >65mmHg with vasopressors.
b.   Transfusing blood early to improve oxygen delivery.
c.   Aiming for a core/peripheral temperature difference of >2°C.
d.   Aiming for a haematocrit of 30% by administering boluses of intravenous fluids.
e.   Routine use of a vasodilator such as hydralazine.

19 The cardiac cycle describes the relationship between the electrical and mechanical events within the heart over time. Which of the following events is most likely to coincide with the second heart sound?

a. Isovolumetric relaxation and the ST segment of the ECG.
b. A rise in atrial pressure and the V wave of jugular venous pressure.
c. The dicrotic notch of the aortic pressure trace and the y descent of the jugular venous pressure.
d. The end of the T wave on the ECG and a fall in atrial pressure.
e. Passive filling of the ventricles and the T wave on the ECG.

20 A 60-year-old male patient presents with a history of crushing central chest pain which started 9 hours ago and lasted for over an hour. Blood tests are taken immediately. Which of the following cardiac enzymes is the most sensitive marker in acute coronary syndrome?

a. Aspartate aminotransferase (AST).
b. Creatine kinase-MB (CK-MB).
c. Lactic dehydrogenase (LDH).
d. Troponin I.
e. Troponin C.

21 A 20-year-old female patient with a recent diagnosis of lymphoma is receiving chemotherapy. Which one of the following would be the most effective regime in the prevention of nausea/vomiting?

a. Metoclopramide 10mg IV and cyclizine 50mg IV.
b. Droperidol 1.25mg IV and prochlorperazine 12.5mg IV.
c. Metoclopramide 10mg IV and ondansetron 8mg IV.
d. Ondansetron 8mg IV and dexamethasone 8mg IV.
e. Prochlorperazine 12.5mg IV and dexamethasone 8mg IV.

22

A 45-year-old man of Afro-Caribbean descent presents with three elevated blood pressure measurements of 165/105 over a 6-week period. Which of the following would be the most appropriate medication to start treatment with?

a. Ramipril.
b. Valsartan.
c. Doxazosin.
d. Carvedilol.
e. Amlodipine.

23

A patient with severe refractory depression is scheduled for a mastectomy due to breast cancer. She is on phenelzine for her depression. What is the most appropriate management regarding her phenelzine?

a. Continue phenelzine to the day of surgery and omit the morning dose.
b. Discontinue phenelzine 2 weeks prior to surgery and start fluoxetine.
c. Discontinue phenelzine 2 weeks prior to surgery, start moclobemide and omit moclobemide on the day of surgery.
d. Discontinue phenelzine 2 weeks prior to surgery.
e. Discontinue phenelzine 2 weeks prior to surgery, start moclobemide and continue till surgery.

24

A 29-year-old female patient with porphyria presents for an emergency laparotomy for a ruptured ectopic pregnancy. Her heart rate is 92/minute and blood pressure is 110/60mmHg. Which one of the following anaesthetic drugs is most unsafe in this patient?

a. Isoflurane.
b. Thiopentone.
c. Propofol.
d. Ketamine.
e. Suxamethonium.

25 A 21-year-old ASA1 patient needs an intravenous infusion of drug A. The following are the available data for drug A: 1) the desired steady-state plasma concentration is 0.2mg/ml; 2) the volume of distribution at steady state is 5000ml; 3) the clearance is 200ml/minute. Which one of the following correctly represents the intravenous loading dose for drug A?

a.   1000mg.
b.   400mg.
c.   200mg.
d.   40mg.
e.   2000mg.

26 A piece of medical monitoring equipment is designed to have a leakage current of less than 50µA and contains a floating circuit. Which of the following classes does this equipment belong to?

a.   Class BF.
b.   Class CF.
c.   Class B.
d.   Class II F.
e.   Class I.

27 A study is conducted to compare the efficacy of 5% hypertonic saline and 20% mannitol in reducing intracranial pressure (ICP) in patients with traumatic brain injury. Mean ICP values are available for two groups before and after the intervention. Assuming that the ICP values are normally distributed (Gaussian distribution), which of the following statistical tests would be most appropriate in comparing the two groups?

a.   Wilcoxon signed rank test.
b.   Student's t-test.
c.   ANOVA paired test.
d.   Paired student's t-test.
e.   Mann-Whitney U test.

28 A 60-year-old male patient is undergoing a craniotomy and blood pressure is being invasively monitored via an arterial cannula inserted through the left radial artery. Half way through the procedure you wish to perform a square wave test (fast flush test) to ensure that the arterial system is optimally damped. Which of the following describes under-damping of the system?

a.   The waveform settles to zero without any oscillations.
b.   The waveform settles to zero after several oscillations.
c.   The waveform settles to zero after 2 or 3 oscillations.
d.   The waveform never settles to zero.
e.   The waveform settles to zero after one oscillation.

29 You are performing an interscalene nerve block using a peripheral nerve locator on a 25-year-old woman with a BMI of 23. Which of the following is the most suitable needle for this block?

a.   A 22G, 50mm long insulated needle.
b.   A 20G, 100mm long insulated needle.
c.   A 22G, 25mm long non-insulated needle with a non-cutting tip.
d.   A 22G, 50mm long insulated needle with a non-cutting tip.
e.   A 22G, 25mm long insulated needle with a non-cutting tip.

30 An electromagnetic radiation has a wavelength of 10^{-9} and frequency of 10^{18} and it is in the ultraviolet spectrum. In which one of the following applications is this electromagnetic radiation most suitable for use?

a.   As an X-ray.
b.   As a LASER.
c.   In an infrared analyser.
d.   In a paging system.
e.   In refractometry.

Set 4 answers

1   Answer: D. Nitrous oxide.

The rate at which a gas reaches equilibrium between the alveoli and capillary blood depends on its reaction with the substances in blood. Nitrous oxide does not react and reaches equilibrium in about 0.1s. The uptake of nitrous oxide is not limited by diffusion but by flow through the capillaries (flow-limited).

Carbon monoxide is taken up by haemoglobin at a high rate and equilibrium is not reached even at the end of 0.75s (diffusion-limited).

Oxygen is intermediate and its transfer is perfusion-limited.

Further reading
1. Ganong WF, Ed. Gas exchange in the lungs. In: *Review of medical physiology*, 22nd ed. New York, USA: McGraw-Hill, 2005; Chapter 34: 660-1.

2   Answer: D. 13.4ml/dL.

The maximum amount of O_2 that can be combined with haemoglobin is called oxygen-carrying capacity. One gram of haemoglobin can combine with 1.39ml O_2. The amount of O_2 combined with Hb can be calculated by the formula:

$$O_2 \text{ bound to Hb} = 1.34 \times Hb \times SpO_2/100$$

Substituting the data given in the above equation:

$$O_2 \text{ bound to Hb} = 1.34 \times 10 \times 100/100 = 13.4\text{ml oxygen/dL.}$$

Further reading

1. West JB. Gas transport by the blood. In: *Respiratory physiology - the essentials*, 7th ed. Baltimore, USA: Lippincott Williams & Wilkins, 2005; Chapter 6: 75-80.

3   Answer: B. Low haemoglobin concentration.

There is a higher incidence of apnoea of prematurity (AOP) following general anaesthesia. Neonates will have a low oxygen reserve and increased O_2 consumption. There are fewer type I muscle fibres (slow contracting and highly oxidative) in the neonatal diaphragm and intercostal muscles which lead to increased respiratory muscle fatigue. All these factors can contribute towards hypoxaemia in preterm neonates.

The haemoglobin concentration is expected to be in the range of 17-18g/dL in neonates.

Further reading

1. Maternal and neonatal physiology. In: *Principles of physiology for the anaesthetist*, 1st ed. Power I, Kam P, Eds. London, UK: Arnold (Hodder Headline Group), 2001; Chapter 14: 358-62.

4   Answer: E. Left lateral spinothalamic tract.

Fibres mediating temperature and pain synapse with the neurons in the dorsal horn. The axons from these neurons cross the midline and ascend in the anterolateral quadrant of the spinal cord (lateral spinothalamic tract). Fibres mediating fine touch and proprioception ascend in the dorsal columns, whereas fibres mediating touch and pressure ascend in the ventral spinothalamic tract.

Further reading

1. Ganong WF, Ed. Cutaneous, deep and visceral sensation. In: *Review of medical physiology*, 22nd ed. New York, USA: McGraw-Hill, 2005; Chapter 7: 138-47.

5 Answer: A. Albumin.

Albumin accounts for 70% of the colloid osmotic pressure. 60% of plasma proteins are made up of albumin and approximately 30 to 40% of the body's total albumin pool is found in the intravascular compartment. Albumin does not diffuse freely through intact vascular endothelium. Hence, it is the major protein providing the colloid osmotic or oncotic pressure that regulates the passage of water and diffusible solutes through the capillaries. Albumin has a negative charge at normal plasma pH and attracts and retains cations, especially Na^+ in the vascular compartment. This is called the Gibbs-Donnan effect. Hence, it exerts a greater osmotic force than can be accounted for solely on the basis of the number of molecules dissolved in the plasma. Albumin also binds a small number of Cl^- ions that increase its negative charge and ability to retain Na^+ ions inside the capillaries. This enhanced osmotic force causes the colloid osmotic pressure to be 50% greater than it would be by protein concentration alone.

Globulins make up 35% of plasma proteins and include carrier proteins, enzymes, complement and immunoglobulins.

Further reading
1. Margarson MP, Soni N. Serum albumin: touchstone or totem? *Anaesthesia* 1998; 53: 789-803.

6 Answer: C. Amiodarone.

One of the side effects of long-term treatment with amiodarone is pneumonitis and pulmonary fibrosis. The risk factors include underlying lung diseases, high dose (400mg/day or more) and recent chest infection such as pneumonia. Pulmonary toxicity can be diagnosed early by serial chest X-rays and lung function tests. Other drugs which can cause pulmonary fibrosis are bleomycin, methotrexate, cyclosporin, cyclophosphamide and nitrofurantoin.

Further reading
1. Brunton LL, Lazo JS, Parker KL, Eds. Antiarrhythmic drugs. In: *Goodman & Gilman's the pharmacological basis of therapeutics,* 11th ed. New York, USA: McGraw-Hill, 2006; Chapter 34: 920-3.

7   Answer: C. Non-ionised form.

Non-invasive delivery of medication through the skin surface to produce systemic effects is known as transdermal delivery. The drug needs to be present in a high concentration within the patch for transdermal delivery to occur. The energy for drug release is derived from the concentration gradient existing between a saturated solution of drug in the delivery system and the much lower concentration in the skin.

Drug movement occurs by diffusion; therefore, transdermal permeation is improved if the drug has the following properties:

◆   High potency ensures that the drug is effective at the lowest dose.
◆   Ionisation makes it much easier for the non-ionic component of the drug to cross the lipophilic membrane.
◆   Molecular weight less than 50Da.
◆   Affinity for both lipophilic and hydrophilic phases. Extreme partitioning characteristics are not conducive to successful drug delivery via the skin.
◆   A low melting point ensures easy release of the drug.
◆   Short half-life.

Further reading
1.   Bajaj S, Whiteman A, Brandner B. Transdermal drug delivery in pain management. *British Journal of Anaesthesia CEACCP* 2011; 11: 39-43.

8   Answer: D. Phenelzine.

Phenelzine is a non-selective irreversible monoamine oxidase inhibitor (MAOI) used in the treatment of severe depression.

Doxazocin is an α-adrenoreceptor blocker used in the treatment of hypertension and prostatic hyperplasia.

Fosinopril is an angiotensin-converting enzyme (ACE) inhibitor, used in the treatment of hypertension.

Supplemental thyroxine is indicated in the treatment of hypopthyroidism. Although increased levels of thyroxine can cause tachycardia and hypertension, in this patent, the interaction between phenelzine and ephedrine is more likely to produce a hypertensive crisis.

Monoamine oxidases are enzymes involved in the breakdown of amine neurotransmitters (serotonin and norepinephrine). They are classified as MAO type A, which has a preference for norepinephrine and serotonin, and MAO type B, which deaminates tyramine and phenylethylamine. It is antagonism of MAO type A which is responsible for the antidepressant effect of these MAOIs.

The most important anaesthetic consideration for patients taking MAOIs relates to the hypertensive crisis following indirectly-acting sympathomimetics and opioids such as pethidine. The metabolism of indirectly-acting sympathomimetics is inhibited, resulting in the potentiation of their action.

Directly-acting sympathomimetics are preferable in the treatment of hypertension. They also should be used with extreme caution as they may cause exaggerated hypertension.

Further reading
1. Peck T, Wong A, Norman E. Anaesthetic implications of psychoactive drugs. *British Journal of Anaesthesia CEACCP* 2010; 10: 177-81.

9   Answer: D. Dipyridamole.

Milrinone, enoximone, dipyridamole and amrinone are phosphodiesterase (PDE) enzyme inhibitors. Drugs which inhibit the action of PDE increase the level of cyclic adenosine phosphate (cAMP) by reducing the breakdown of cAMP. There are a number of iso-enzymes of the PDE enzyme. The effect of the action of the inhibitors depends on the iso-enzyme they inhibit.

Milrinone and amrinone act by inhibiting the PDE iso-enzyme 3, which is mainly present in the heart. Enoximone inhibits the PDE iso-enzyme 4 and possibly iso-enzyme 3, present in the heart and vascular smooth muscles.

The clinical effects of milrinone and enoximone are similar. Both are used in the treatment of heart failure.

Dipyridamole acts mainly by inhibiting the PDE iso-enzyme 5, which is present in platelets.

Clopidogrel is an antiplatelet drug and acts by inhibiting adenosine diphosphate binding to its receptor on the platelet surface.

Further reading
1. Feneck R. Phosphodiesterase inhibitors and the cardiovascular system. *British Journal of Anaesthesia CEACCP* 2007; 7: 203-7.

10 Answer: B. PaCO$_2$ of 2.9kPa.

Aspirin (salicylate) is a non-steroidal anti-inflammatory drug (NSAID). In overdose, patients are typically conscious. Symptoms include nausea and vomiting, tinnitus, sweating and confusion. It directly stimulates the respiratory centre resulting in hyperventilation and respiratory alkalosis. The urine is initially alkaline due to bicarbonate excretion which compensates for the respiratory alkalosis. Following the loss of large amounts of urine, dehydration and hypokalaemia develops. A paradoxical aciduria then develops as the kidneys retain potassium in exchange for hydrogen ions.

A metabolic acidosis may also result in the later stages of poisoning due to increased lactate and ketone body production following the uncoupling of oxidative phosphorylation.

Further reading
1. Ward C, Sair M. Oral poisoning: an update. *British Journal of Anaesthesia CEACCP* 2010; 10: 6-11.

11 Answer: C. Use of only CO_2 as insufflation gas during laparoscopic surgery.

Precautions to be taken to minimize the risk of fire and explosions in the operating theatre include:

- Avoidance of use of flammable agents in the operating room.
- Use of spark-free switches.
- Adequate air conditioning and scavenging with 15-20 changes of air per hour in the operating theatre.
- Maintaining a relative humidity of more than 50% in the operating theatre. A dry atmosphere promotes the generation of static electrical charges. However, working in an atmosphere with very high humidity (>80%) is quite uncomfortable.
- Preferable use of circle systems.
- Ensuring that flammable skin preparation solutions have evaporated completely before using the diathermy.
- Avoidance of build-up of static electricity.

The components of a fire triangle include an ignition source, fuel and an oxidizing agent to support combustion.

Static electricity is a known source of ignition in theatre. Materials that are likely to cause static charges such as nylon and wool should be avoided in the theatre environment. Bowel gas contains methane (up to 30%) and hydrogen (up to 44%) which are highly flammable. Liberation of these gases from accidental perforation of the bowel could potentially cause ignition in the abdomen during surgery. Only 100% CO_2 should be used for gas insufflation during laparoscopy. Although the oxygen concentration in the intestines is low (less than 5%) and cannot support a fire, diffusion of nitrous oxide into the bowel and peritoneal cavity poses a potential danger.

The zone of risk is the area of the operating room in which mixtures of anaesthetic agents may be explosive. It extends to 25cm from any part of the anaesthetic apparatus or the patient's airway containing the anaesthetic mixture. Any flame or potential source of risk must be outside this zone.

Further reading
1. Litt L. Electrical safety in the operating room. In: *Miller's anesthesia*, Volume 2, 7th ed. Miller RD, Ed. Philadelphia, USA: Churchill Livingstone, Elsevier, 2010; Chapter 100: 3041-52.
2. Ashman MN, Mathasko MJ. Electrical and fire safety in the operating room. *Seminars in Anesthesia* 1993; 12: 276-81.

12 Answer: C. The volume of the drain tube should be more than 50% of the patient's maximal inspiratory volume.

An underwater seal is used to allow air to escape through the drain but not to re-enter the pleural cavity. The drainage bottle should always be kept below the level of the patient, otherwise its contents will siphon back into the pleural cavity. It should be kept at least 45cm below the level of the patient's chest.

The diameter of the tube should be wide enough to minimise the resistance. The tube from the patient to the drain system must have a volume of more than 50% of the patient's maximum inspiratory volume, or water may be aspirated into the chest during deep inspiration.

The end of the tube within the drain bottle should not be more than 5cm below the surface of the water as it increases the resistance for the air to escape. The total volume of the water in the bottle should be more than the volume of the drainage tube to prevent in-drawing of air during inspiration. Suction should only be used for a non-resolving pneumothorax and should not exceed more than -20cm H_2O.

Further reading
1. Kam AC, O'Brien M, Kam PCA. Pleural drainage systems. *Anaesthesia* 1993; 48: 154-61.
2. Laws D, Neville E, Duffy J. BTS Guidelines for the insertion of a chest drain. *Thorax* 2003; 58: ii53.
3. Etoch SW, Bar-Natan MF, Miller FB, Richardson JD. Tube thoracostomy. Factors relating to complications. *Archives of Surgery* 1995; 130: 521-5.

13 Answer: D. Immersion in 2% glutaraldehyde solution.

A fibreoptic endoscope can be effectively disinfected with glutaraldehyde 2%. Glutaraldehyde is non-corrosive and does not damage the lens or the fibreoptic bundles of the scope. It is an irritant to the eyes, skin and mucous membranes. It is effective against bacteria, mycobacteria, viruses and spores.

Formaldehyde is a highly toxic and flammable gas that has been used as a disinfectant and a sterilant in both a water-based solution (formalin) and in the gaseous state. Its uses are limited by its pungent odour and fumes, which irritate the skin, eyes, and respiratory tract.

Ethylene oxide is a colourless, flammable gas. The gas is penetrative and non-corrosive. In particular it is used to sterilize single-use medical items that would be damaged by the excessive heat used in other sterilization methods. Disadvantages of ethylene oxide are that it is toxic and long periods of aeration are required after sterilisation.

Quaternary ammonium compounds are low-level disinfectants. They are bactericidal, fungicidal, and virucidal but do not have sporicidal effects.

Fibreoptic scopes cannot be steam sterilised as the temperature would damage the fibreoptic bundles and coating.

Further reading
1. Dorsch JA, Dorsch SE. Cleaning and sterilization. In: *Understanding anesthesia equipment*, 5th ed. New York, USA: Lippincott Williams & Wilkins, 2007; Chapter 34: 958-90.

14 Answer: C. Dead space gas is re-used.

Although all statements are correct, the most important reason is that the dead space gas is re-used. In a Mapelson A system, the spill valve (adjustable pressure relief valve) is located at the patient end and the reservoir bag at the machine end. During the initial part of expiration the dead space gas, which does not contain CO_2, flows backwards towards the reservoir bag. The reservoir bag continues to fill with fresh gas flow. Once it is full the spill valve opens and alveolar gas containing CO_2 from the patient is exhaled.

Further reading
1. Mapleson WW. Anaesthetic breathing systems. *British Journal of Anaesthesia CEACCP* 2001; 1: 3-7.

15 Answer: C. It is double insulated equipment and the earth wire is not essential.

To ensure safety and prevent electrical hazards, all medical equipment should meet the requirement of certain national and international standards. IEC (international electronic commission) 60601-1, introduced in 2005, describes the general requirements for basic safety and essential performance of medical equipment.

Medical monitoring equipment is classified according to the means of protection against electrical shock:

- Class 1: any conducting part of the equipment, which may contact the patient, is connected to earth by an earth wire. It incorporates a fuse in the mains plug that melts to break the circuit when a live supply comes into contact with the accessible part, and it also has a fuse in the live and neutral conductors for additional protection.
- Class 2: this has a double insulation or reinforced insulation. An earth wire is not required.
- Class 3: this is battery-powered equipment with a voltage not exceeding 25V AC or 60V DC. Even with this low voltage, the risk of microshock still exists.

Further reading
1. Kadavil HP, Palmer J. Electrical hazards: causes and prevention. *Anaesthesia and Intensive Care Medicine* 2011; 11: 458-60.
2. Boumphrey S, Langton JA. Electrical safety in the operating theatre. *British Journal of Anaesthesia CEACCP* 2003; 3: 10-4.

16 Answer: A. It replaces nitrogen in the FRC with oxygen.

Pre-oxygenation replaces nitrogen in the functional residual capacity (FRC) with oxygen (denitrogenation of the FRC). The FRC is the most important store of oxygen in the body. A longer period of apnoea can be tolerated if there is an increased oxygen store in the FRC, thus delaying critical hypoxia.

Pre-oxygenation does increase the inspired oxygen concentration, which increases the partial pressure of oxygen in the alveolus. It also increases the dissolved oxygen in blood, but this is not clinically significant. Pre-oxygenation does not affect the shunt fraction.

123

Further reading
1. Sirian R, Wills JI. Physiology of apnoea and the benefits of preoxygenation. *British Journal of Anaesthesia CEACCP* 2009; 9: 105-8.

17 Answer: D. Reduced FRC due to supine position and general anaesthesia.

The normal functional residual capacity (FRC) is approximately 30ml/kg, about 2100ml in a 70kg male. In elderly patients, the closing capacity increases, nearing functional residual capacity even in a sitting position. If the closing capacity exceeds the FRC, small airway closure will occur. Therefore, they are more prone to airway collapse, increasing ventilation/perfusion mismatch and hypoxia. The response to hypercarbia and hypoxia is blunted in elderly patients. The FRC is reduced by up to 1000ml when the supine position is adopted, due to the abdominal contents shifting towards the chest. During general anaesthesia, the FRC is reduced both during controlled and spontaneous ventilation. In obese patients, this reduction in FRC is more pronounced.

Absorption atelectasis can occur particularly in alveoli with low V/Q units when a FiO_2 of 1.0 is used.

Further reading
1. Lumb AB, Ed. Changes in functional residual capacity. In: *Nunn's applied respiratory physiology*, 7th ed. Philadelphia, USA: Churchill Livingstone, Elsevier 2010; Chapter 22: 333-7.
2. Wilson WC, Benumof JL. Respiratory function during anaesthesia. In: *Miller's anesthesia*, Volume 1, 7th ed. Miller RD, Ed. Philadelphia, USA: Churchill Livingstone, Elsevier, 2010; Chapter 17: 705-18.

18 Answer: D. Aiming for a haematocrit of 30% by administering boluses of intravenous fluids.

For free flap survival, blood flow through the microvasculature must be maximized. This is best achieved by maintaining laminar flow. According to the principles of the Hagen Poiseuille equation, the flow rate is directly proportional to the driving pressure, the radius to the power 4, and inversely proportional to the viscosity of the blood. Therefore, the best flap perfusion is achieved by maintaining a good cardiac output, maintaining the haematocrit around 30% and by avoiding hypothermia and vasoconstriction. At a haematocrit >40%, viscosity increases dramatically.

Although a MAP of >65mm Hg is essential, using vasopressors may cause vasoconstriction and reduce the blood flow. The core and peripheral temperature difference should be maintained at less than 2°C. Adequate vasodilation is usually achieved with anaesthetic agents.

Further reading
1. Quinlan J, Lodi O. Anaesthesia for reconstructive surgery. *Anaesthesia and Intensive Care Medicine* 2009; 10: 26-31.

19 Answer: B. A rise in atrial pressure and the V wave of jugular venous pressure.

The second heart sound (closure of the aortic and pulmonary valves) hails the onset of diastole. It occurs at the beginning of phase 4 (isovolumetric relaxation), which follows the end of the T wave on the ECG. It coincides with the dicrotic notch on the aortic trace, isovolumetric relaxation of the ventricle and the V wave of the CVP trace. Following isovolumetric relaxation, the mitral and tricuspid valves open and ventricular filling begins.

During isovolumetric relaxation, the ventricles relax as a closed cavity and the pressure in the ventricles continues to drop. When the pressure within the ventricle drops below the atrial pressure, ventricular filling begins.

The ST segment on the ECG corresponds to ventricular systole. The ST segment and T wave are both produced by ventricular repolarization.

The first heart sound is produced by the vibrations set up by the closure of the mitral and tricuspid valves.

The second heart sound is caused by the vibrations associated with closure of the aortic and pulmonary valves.

The third heard sound is produced by rapid ventricular filling.

A fourth heart sound can sometimes be heard immediately before the first heart sound. This is produced by atrial contraction resulting in rapid flow of blood from the atria to the ventricles.

Further reading
1. Ganong WF, Ed. Mechanical events of the cardiac cycle. In: *Review of medical physiology*, 22nd ed. New York, USA: McGraw-Hill, 2005: 565-70.

20 Answer: D. Troponin I.

Many enzymes are released trom within cardiac cells into the blood following an acute injury.

A cardiospecific isoform of creatinine kinase (CK-MB) starts to rise 4-6 hours after myocardial injury and peaks at about 12 hours. Creatinine kinase levels also increase following skeletal muscle injury and defibrillation. Troponin T and I are the most sensitive markers. They are released within 4-6 hours and remain elevated for up to 2 weeks.

Normally cardiac troponins are not detectable. Monoclonoal antibody tests for cardiac-specific troponin I and cardiac-specific troponin T are highly sensitive markers of myocyte necrosis. Troponin I has a 90% sensitivity and 95% specificity for myocardial infarction 8 hours after the onset of symptoms and troponin T has an 84% sensitivity and 81% specificity for myocardial infarction 8 hours after the onset of symptoms. Both these enzymes rise 3-6 hours after onset of symptoms and peak at about 20 hours.

Further reading
1. Bloomfield P, Bradbury A, Brubb NR, Newby DE. In: *Davidson's principles and practice of medicine*, 20th ed. Boon NA, Colledge NR, Walker BR, Hunter JAA, Eds. Churchill Livingstone, Elsevier, 2006; Chapter 18: 591-4.

21 Answer: D. Ondansetron 8mg IV and dexamethasone 8mg IV.

Ondansetron is a 5HT3 antagonist used both for the prophylaxis and treatment of postoperative nausea and vomiting (PONV). It is particularly useful in the treatment of nausea and vomiting associated with chemotherapy and radiotherapy.

Dexamethasone is also used in the treatment of nausea and vomiting associated with chemotherapy. A combination of dexamethasone (8-10mg IV) and ondansetron (8mg IV) is indicated as prophylaxis for moderate to high emetogenic chemotherapy.

Cyclizine is used as an anti-emetic in treating PONV associated with opioids and in motion sickness.

Metoclopramide is a prokinetic agent and is less effective in treating PONV when compared to other anti-emetics such as 5HT3 antagonists and anti-histamines.

Prochlorperazine is a dopamine antagonist effective in the prevention of PONV.

Further reading
1. Peck TE, Hill SA, Williams M, Eds. Anti-emetics and related drugs. In: *Pharmacology for anaesthesia and intensive care*, 3rd ed. Cambridge, UK: Cambridge University Press, 2008; Chapter 18: 282-91.

22 Answer: E. Amlodipine.

Amlodipine is a calcium channel blocker with a half-life of 40 hours. It is suitable for once daily administration. If blood pressure over 160/105 persists over a 4-12 week period or if target organ damage or diabetes is present, treatment should be instituted. First-line therapy in a patient 55 years or older or a black patient of any age is a calcium channel blocker or thiazide-type diuretic. In all other younger patients the treatment of choice is an angiotensin-converting enzyme (ACE) inhibitor. Second-line therapy for all groups is a combination of an ACE inhibitor and a calcium channel blocker or an ACE inhibitor and a thiazide-type diuretic. Third-line management is a combination of all three.

Ramipril is an ACE inhibitor and is not suitable for first-line therapy in this patient. Valsartan is an angiotensin-II receptor antagonist with properties similar to ACE inhibitors. Doxazosin blocks the post-synaptic α-1 adrenoreceptors and produces vasodilatation. Carvedilol is a β-blocker and arteriolar dilator, particularly reducing peripheral vascular resistance.

Further reading
1. Williams B, Poulter NR, Brown MJ, *et al.* British Hypertension Society guidelines for hypertension management 2004. *British Medical Journal* 2004; 328: 634-40.

23 Answer: C. Discontinue phenelzine 2 weeks prior to surgery, start moclobemide and omit moclobemide on the day of surgery.

A patient on an MAOI (monoamine oxidase inhibitor) is a clear indication that the psychiatric treatment has had a complicated course and that conventional therapy was unsuccessful. Abrupt discontinuation of the

MAOI can result in severe withdrawal symptoms or disease recurrence presenting with severe depression, delusions and hallucinations.

MAOIs can be involved in serious life-threatening interactions with sympathomimetics (especially the indirectly-acting sympathomimetics), nefopam and opioid analgesia (especially pethidine). Therefore, consideration should be given to decide whether to continue or discontinue the drug. The consequences of these interactions are two-fold: firstly, significant hypertension due to the release of intracellular stores of norepinephrine and epinephrine and, secondly, a CNS effect due to serotonergic over-activity.

There are irreversible MAOIs (phenelzine and tranylcypromine) and reversible MAOIs (moclobemide). With irreversible inhibitors it takes 1-4 weeks for the enzyme to regain activity and with reversible MAOIs the effects are reversed within 16 hours.

It is recommended that in the instance where an irreversible MAOI is used, that the drug is discontinued 2 weeks prior to surgery and a reversible MAOI started with the dose being omitted on the day of surgery.

In an emergency when there is no time to discontinue the irreversible MAOI, the anaesthetist needs to avoid pethidine and only use directly-acting sympathomimetics with extreme caution.

Fluoxetine is a selective serotonin-reuptake inhibitor (SSRI) and is less likely to be successful in controlling symptoms in this patient.

Further reading
1. Peck T, Wong A, Norman E. Anaesthetic implications of psychoactive drugs. *British Journal of Anaesthesia CEACCP* 2010; 10: 177-81.
2. Huyse FJ, Touw DJ, *et al.* Psychotropic drugs and the perioperative period: a proposal for a guideline in elective surgery. *Psychosomatics* 2006; 47: 8-22.

24 Answer: B. Thiopentone.

This patient has porphyria, which restricts the choices of drugs which can be used in an emergency. Barbiturates (thiopentone, methohexitone) are definitely unsafe. Judicious use of propofol (along with boluses or infusion of vasopressors) would be the preferred drug for induction. As this patient requires rapid sequence induction and there is no contraindication for using suxamethonium, it can be used. Ketamine is probably safe and is unlikely to provoke acute porphyria. Similarly volatile agents such as isoflurane have been used safely in patients with porphyria.

Further reading

1. Grant IS, Nimmo GR, Nimmo S. Intercurrent disease and anaesthesia. In: *Textbook of anaesthesia*, 5th ed. Aitkenhead AR, Smith G, Rowbotham DJ. Eds: Philadelphia, USA: Churchill Livingstone, Elsevier, 2006; Chapter 23: 482-3.
2. Stoelting RK, Dierdorf SF. Inborn errors of metabolism. In: *Anesthesia and co-existing disease*, 4th ed. Philadelphia, USA: Churchill Livingstone, 2002: 455-70.

25 Answer: A. 1000mg.

When a drug is administered intravenously, dosage regimens can be used to produce accurate and constant plasma concentrations.

The required loading dose in milligrams is calculated by the equation:

$$Cp \times V$$

and the rate of infusion is calculated by the equation:

$$Cp \times CL$$

Where Cp = the desired steady-state plasma concentration required to produce a given effect (mg/ml); CL = the clearance of a drug (ml/min); V = volume of distribution at steady state.

Further reading

1. Calvey TN, Williams NE. Pharmacokinetics. In: *Principles and practice of pharmacology for anaesthetists*, 4th ed. Oxford, UK: Blackwell Science, 2001; Chapter 2: 24-5.

26   Answer: B. Class CF.

Medical monitoring equipment is classified according to the maximum leakage currents permissible for a particular application. Equipment with electrodes that may contact the heart directly is termed type CF, indicating it is for cardiac use and has a floating circuit. The leakage current allowed for CF equipment is less than 50μA. For type B or BF equipment, the maximum leakage current is less than 500μA.

Further reading

1. Davis PD, Kenny GNC, Eds. Electrical safety. In: *Basic physics and measurement in anaesthesia*, 5th ed. London, UK: Butterworth Heinemann, 2003; Chapter 16: 179-86.

27   Answer: D. Paired student's t-test.

A student's t-test is most commonly used when comparing data from two normally distributed samples. It calculates t, using the formula:

$$t = \frac{\text{Difference between means}}{\text{Standard error of difference}}$$

Data in the above study can be considered as paired since the variables under test are from the same patient. The ICP is measured before and after the intervention (saline or mannitol), hence, these measurements are paired. Since the data are normally distributed, a paired student's t-test is the appropriate statistical test to be used for this study. Paired statistical tests are sensitive and require fewer patients in each group to achieve statistical significance.

If the data are not distributed normally, a Wilcoxon signed rank test may be used for paired data and the Mann-Whitney U test for unpaired data.

The Mann-Whitney U test is a non-parametric test that can be used in place of an unpaired t-test. It is used to test the null hypothesis that two samples come from the same population (i.e. have the same median) or, alternatively, whether observations in one sample tend to be larger than observations in the other.

An ANOVA test is used for normally distributed data where more than two groups are involved in the study.

Further reading

1. Rowbotham DJ. Basic statistics. In: *Fundamentals of anaesthesia*, 3rd ed. Pinnock C, Lin T, Smith T, Eds. Cambridge, UK: Cambridge University Press, 2009; Section 2, Chapter 14: 485-98.

28 Answer: B. The waveform settles to zero after several oscillations.

To determine the optimum damping of the system a square wave test (fast flush test) is used.

To perform the square wave test the system is flushed by applying a pressure of 300mm Hg (the flush button is compressed and released or the lever located near the transducer is pulled). This results in a square waveform followed by oscillations.

In an optimally damped system, there will be two or three oscillations before settling to zero. An over-damped system settles to zero without any oscillations. In an under-damped system, the waveform settles to zero after several oscillations.

The damping coefficient indicates how fast the oscillating system will come to rest.

If the damping coefficient = 0, then there is no damping, so oscillation will continue indefinitely.

If the damping coefficient =1 (critically damped), there is just enough damping to prevent oscillations.

For a fluid-filled catheter system, a damping coefficient = 0.67 is considered as optimal damping.

Further reading
1. Bedford RF, Shah NK. Blood pressure monitoring. In: *Monitoring in anaesthesia and critical care*, 3rd ed. Blitt CD, Hines RL, Eds. New York, USA: Churchill Livingstone, 1995: 95-130.

29 Answer: E. 22G, 25mm long insulated needle with a non-cutting tip.

Purpose designed thin insulated needles are used in conjunction with the nerve locator to precisely locate the nerve. When a non-insulated needle is used, the current disperses in all directions and, hence, a larger current is needed to stimulate the nerve. In this patient (with a BMI of 23), the brachial plexus is superficial in the interscalene groove. Therefore, a needle longer than 25mm is unnecessary. A non-cutting needle reduces the chance of nerve damage. A larger diameter needle can increase the risk of tissue damage. Hence, a 22G, 25mm insulated needle is preferred in this scenario.

Further reading
1. Dalrymple P, Chelliah S. Electrical nerve locators. *British Journal of Anaesthesia CEACCP* 2006; 6: 32-6.

30 Answer: A. As an X ray.

In a spectrum of electromagnetic radiation used in medicine, X-rays and gamma rays have the highest frequency (10^{18} to 10^{21}Hz) and shortest wavelength (10^{-9} to 10^{-12}). These rays are in the ultraviolet spectrum. The electromagnetic radiation used in infrared red analysers and paging systems are in the infrared light spectrum, which has the longest wavelength and lowest frequency. Visible light radiation is used in a LASER and refractometer.

Set 5 questions

1   The chemoreceptors in the carotid body detect changes in the composition of blood to activate the respiratory centre in the medulla. Which one of the following changes leads to the greatest stimulation of carotid body chemoreceptors?

a.   Oxygen saturation of haemoglobin.
b.   Partial pressure of oxygen.
c.   Oxygen content of blood.
d.   pH of blood.
e.   Partial pressure of CO_2.

2   Urea plays an important role in the counter-current mechanism in the kidney. In which part of the nephron is urea reabsorbed maximally?

a.   Proximal tubule in the cortex.
b.   Distal tubule in the cortex.
c.   Collecting duct.
d.   Proximal tubule in the medulla.
e.   Distal tubule in the medulla.

3   During the cardiac cycle, which one of the following leads to most of the ventricular filling?

a.   Atrial electrical systole.
b.   Passive flow of the blood from atrium to ventricle.
c.   Atrial mechanical systole.
d.   Rise in pulmonary artery pressure.
e.   Drop in intrathoracic pressure.

4   Calcium homeostasis is essential for normal function of the human body. Which one of the following has the most important role in the regulation of the serum calcium level?

a.   Active vitamin D.
b.   Parathyroid hormone.
c.   Calcitonin.
d.   Renal tubular absorption.
e.   Dietary calcium level.

5   Which one of the following statements on the composition of cerebrospinal fluid (CSF) is most accurate?

a.   The partial pressure of CO_2 is 42mmHg.
b.   Concentration of protein is very low as compared to that in plasma.
c.   Glucose concentration is the same as that in plasma.
d.   The pH of CSF is slightly higher than 7.4.
e.   Cholesterol concentration is higher than that in plasma.

6   A 64-year-old woman is admitted to intensive care with severe septicaemia. She is treated with a multitude of antibiotics. A few days later she develops diarrhoea and the stool sample analysis confirms *Clostridium difficile* infection. Which one of the following would be the most appropriate in the treatment of diarrhoea?

a.   Intravenous clarithromycin.
b.   Oral metronidazole.
c.   Intravenous metronidazole.
d.   Oral vancomycin.
e.   Intravenous teicoplanin.

7   A 32-year-old male is admitted to intensive care following a severe chest infection. He is intubated and ventilated. He is sedated with an intravenous infusion of propofol and to facilitate positive pressure ventilation, an atracurium infusion was started 12 hours ago. His other medications include rifampicin, amoxicillin and clarithromycin. A few days later his urine appeared greenish. Which of the following is the most likely cause for urine discolouration?

a.   Atracurium infusion.
b.   Sepsis.
c.   Propofol infusion.
d.   Severe septicaemia.
e.   Rifampicin.

8   A 26-year-old lady had an epidural analgesia for labour. She has a past history of cardiac arrhythmias; however, pregnancy has been uneventful. Following delivery she complains of severe headache, which is relieved on lying down. Which one of the following would be the most appropriate next step in the management of headache?

a.   Epidural blood patch.
b.   Oral fluids and paracetamol.
c.   Synthetic ACTH.
d.   Caffeine 300mg.
e.   Desmopressin 4g.

9   A 40-year-old male is admitted to coronary care following a history of palpitations and syncope. On admission, his heart rate is 140/minute and blood pressure is 110/78mmHg. A twelve-lead

Single Best Answer MCQs in Anaesthesia

ECG shows regular narrow complex tachycardia. P waves are clearly noted on the ECG. Carotid sinus massage and adenosine 6mg have been tried, with failure to control the heart rate. Which one of the following would be the most appropriate next step in management?

a. Verapamil 10mg IV.
b. Repeat adenosine 6mg IV.
c. Amiodarone 300mg IV.
d. Repeat adenosine 12mg IV.
e. Electrical cardioversion.

10 A 34-year-old man weighing 96kg has undergone an appendicectomy. He has been prescribed oral morphine for postoperative pain relief on the ward. Considering the bioavailability of morphine, which one of the following would be the effective dose at target site after oral ingestion of 10mg morphine?

a. 1mg of morphine.
b. 3mg of morphine.
c. 6mg of morphine.
d. 5mg of morphine.
e. 10mg of morphine.

11 A 78-year-old patient, weighing 68kg is anaesthetised for a hernia repair. He is breathing spontaneously through a laryngeal mask airway. Anaesthesia is maintained with 1.5 MAC of isoflurane and nitrous oxide (60%) and oxygen (40%) using a fresh gas flow of 0.8L/ minute. Analgesia is provided with incremental boluses of fentanyl. His heart rate is 58 bpm, oxygen saturation is 95% and $EtCO_2$ is 8kPa. Which of the following is the most likely cause for the raised $EtCO_2$?

a. Malignant hyperthermia.
b. Exhausted sodalime.
c. Malfunction of inspiratory unidirectional valve of circle system.
d. Malfunction of expiratory unidirectional valve of circle system.
e. Hypoventilation.

12 A 45-year-old male patient is undergoing a mastoidectomy under general anaesthesia. He is ventilated using a circle absorber system and low-flow anaesthesia. Which of the following is the single most important factor in preventing a critical incident related to a breathing system disconnection?

a. Pulse oximeter.
b. Capnography.
c. Electronic airway pressure monitor.
d. Vigilant anaesthetist continuously monitoring chest wall excursion.
e. Spirometry.

13 A 56-year-old female patient is scheduled for a posterior fossa craniotomy in the sitting position. Which of the following is the most sensitive monitor in detecting intra-operative venous air embolism?

a. Oesophageal stethoscope.
b. Transoesophageal echocardiography.
c. Right atrial pressure monitoring.
d. Precordial Doppler.
e. End-tidal CO_2 monitoring.

14 You are planning to administer a volatile anaesthetic using a completely closed breathing system where all the exhaled gases are re-breathed after absorption of CO_2. Which of the following monitoring is the most essential?

a. Monitoring inspired oxygen concentration using a fuel cell at the common gas outlet.
b. Monitoring inspired oxygen concentration very close to the endotracheal tube.
c. Monitoring inspired CO_2 concentration to detect hypercapnia.
d. Monitoring inspired concentration of volatile anaesthetic agent at the common gas outlet.
e. Monitoring end-tidal CO_2 concentration.

15 A 50-year-old male patient is ready to be transferred from a district general hospital to a neurosurgical centre by ambulance. He is mechanically ventilated to achieve a minute volume of 5L/minute, using a portable ventilator, which consumes 5L/minute of oxygen to drive the ventilator. The total journey time is about 45 minutes. The ventilator requires 20 bar of pressure to operate. How many E-sized oxygen cylinders would be needed to complete the journey?

a. One.
b. Two.
c. Three.
d. Four.
e. Five.

16 Narcosis due to deep sea diving is a well-known phenomenon. Which one of the following gases is least likely to cause narcosis during deep sea diving?

a. Nitrogen.
b. Oxygen.
c. Neon.
d. Carbon dioxide.
e. Helium.

17 The hepatic acinus is roughly divided into three zones that correspond to distance from the arterial blood supply. Which of the following zones is likely to be damaged as a result of paracetamol overdose?

a. Zone 1.
b. Zone 2.
c. Zone 3.
d. All zones.
e. Zone 1 and zone 3 only.

18 As part of human thermoregulation, at an environmental temperature of 39°C, which one of the following is the most effective process in maintaining normal body temperature?

a.   Radiation.
b.   Conduction.
c.   Convection.
d.   Evaporation.
e.   Radiation and convection.

19 A number of factors affect cerebral blood flow. In which of the following factors will a small change (in percentage terms) result in the greatest change in cerebral blood flow?

a.   Partial pressure of oxygen.
b.   Partial pressure of CO_2.
c.   Intracranial pressure.
d.   Body temperature.
e.   Blood pressure.

20 Blood pressure regulation is multi-factorial. Which one of the following is the least likely to cause sustained hypertension in a 41-year-old female?

a.   Long-term use of oral contraceptives.
b.   Sustained increase in the secretion of hormones in the zona glomerulosa in the adrenal cortex.
c.   Sustained increase in the secretion of hormones in the zona fasciculata and zona reticularis in the adrenal cortex.
d.   Sustained increase in the secretion of hormones in the posterior pituitary gland.
e.   Sustained increase in the secretion of hormones in the adrenal medulla.

21 A 72-year-old male is listed for a laparoscopic cholecystectomy. He has severe rheumatoid arthritis, well-controlled atrial fibrillation and polymyalgia rheumatica. He has been on amiodarone, methotrexate, simvastatin and leflunomide for the last 12 years. On the basis of the above information, which one of the following would be the most appropriate pre-operative investigation?

a.   Transoesophageal echocardiogram.
b.   Pulmonary function tests.
c.   Coagulation screen.
d.   Electromyogram.
e.   Muscle biopsy.

22 A 40-year-old male is due to undergo a maxillary reconstruction procedure. During induction of general anaesthesia, thiopentone is accidentally injected into the arterial cannula port. This is noticed immediately and further injection stopped. 4ml of 2.5% thiopentone has been injected through the arterial cannula. What should be the most appropriate next step in managing this situation?

a.   Leave the arterial line *in situ*, inject procaine and perform a stellate ganglion block.
b.   Leave the arterial line *in situ*, administer intravenous heparin and perform a stellate ganglion block.
c.   Leave the arterial line *in situ*, administer a therapeutic dose of LMWH and postpone surgery.
d.   Flush the cannula with heparin, and remove immediately.
e.   Flush the cannula with saline, remove immediately, and perform a stellate ganglion block.

23 A 42-year-old male with severe pneumonia is intubated and ventilated for more than a week in the intensive care unit. He has now been transferred to the operating theatre for placement of a nasojejunal tube under endoscopic guidance in view of establishing enteral feeding. Which one of the following would be the most appropriate drug to facilitate enteral feeding?

a. Prochlorperazine.
b. Erythromycin.
c. Dexamethasone.
d. Cyclizine.
e. Ondansetron.

24 A 28-year-old gravida 4 para 3 is undergoing a category 2 Caesarean section. The baby has been delivered, two boluses of oxytocin 5U have already been administered followed by an infusion of 40U of oxytocin in 500ml normal saline at 125ml/hour. The obstetrician says the uterine tone is poor. Which one of the following would be the most appropriate step?

a. 20U oxytocin intravenous bolus.
b. Inhaled salbutamol.
c. Intramuscular oxytocin and ergometrine.
d. Intravenous prostaglandin F.
e. Intravenous prostaglandin E.

25 A 79-year-old male patient with type 2 diabetes and chronic renal impairment is scheduled for incision and drainage of a peri-anal abscess. His regular medication includes enalapril, spironolactone, gliclazide and simvastatin. On the ward he has been prescribed diclofenac and co-codamol for his pain. On investigating his renal parameters, which one of the following electrolyte abnormalities is most likely to present?

a. Hyperkalaemia.
b. Hypokalaemia.
c. Hypernatraemia.
d. Hypomagnesaemia.
e. Hypocalcaemia.

26 A 76-year-old female patient with ischaemic heart disease is undergoing a laparotomy for a small bowel resection. Invasive arterial blood pressure is being monitored through a 20-gauge arterial cannula in the left radial artery. The transducer system is secured on a drip stand and zeroed with reference to the mid-axillary point. On request from the surgeon, the table is lowered by 10cm and the recorded mean arterial pressure (MAP) is 70mmHg. Which of the following is the true blood pressure at this time?

a.   75mmHg.
b.   80mmHg.
c.   60mmHg.
d   62.4mmHg.
e.   77.6mmHg.

27 Which of the following is the most common complication of direct laryngoscopy and tracheal intubation?

a.   Dental trauma.
b.   Oesophageal intubation.
c.   Pulmonary aspiration.
d.   Subglottic stenosis.
e.   Laryngospasm.

28 Which of the following properties of ultrasound is most useful in diagnostic imaging techniques?

a.   Frequency of ultrasound wave.
b.   Speed of propagation of ultrasound wave.
c.   Absorption of ultrasound by tissues.
d.   Reflection of ultrasound beam at tissue interfaces.
e.   Wavelength of ultrasound wave.

29 During an elective ophthalmic procedure you have been using an atracurium infusion with neuromuscular monitoring. At the end of the procedure, which of the following train-of-four (TOF) responses best suggests administration of neostigmine and glycopyrrolate for reversing the block?

a. One twitch on TOF stimulation.
b. Two twitches on TOF stimulation.
c. Train-of-four ratio >0.4.
d. Four twitches on TOF response.
e. Three twitches on TOF response.

30 A 67-year-old male patient is undergoing a total hip replacement under general anaesthesia. The airway is secured with a tracheal tube, and anaesthesia is maintained with sevoflurane (3%) and nitrous oxide (60%), and oxygen (40%) using a fresh gas flow of 0.3L/minute. Although the sevoflurane dial is set at 3%, the agent analyser indicates an inspired sevoflurane concentration of 1.8%. Which of the following is the most appropriate explanation for the difference between the dial setting and the inspired concentration?

a. Malfunctioning vaporiser.
b. Malfunctioning agent analyser.
c. Ventilator malfunction.
d. Increased uptake of volatile agent by the patient.
e. The dilutional effect of rebreathing.

Set 5 answers

1   Answer: B. Partial pressure of oxygen.

The carotid body is a small cluster of chemoreceptors located near the bifurcation of the carotid artery. The carotid body detects changes in the composition of arterial blood flowing through it, mainly the partial pressure of oxygen, but also of CO_2, pH, and temperature.

The carotid body contains the most vascular tissue in the human body (the rate of blood flow is 2L/100g/minute) and functions as a sensor. It responds to a stimulus, primarily the partial pressure of oxygen, which is detected by type I (glomus) cells, and triggers an action potential in an afferent nerve fibre, the carotid sinus nerve, which relays the information to the central nervous system.

The carotid body also senses increases in the partial pressure of CO_2 and decreases in arterial pH, but to a lesser degree than for partial pressure of oxygen.

The output of carotid bodies is low at an oxygen partial pressure above approximately 100mmHg (13.3kPa), but below this the activity of type I cells increases rapidly. They contain oxygen-sensitive potassium channels, whose conductance is reduced proportional to the degree of hypoxia to which they are exposed. This reduces potassium efflux and causes calcium influx via L-type calcium channels. The calcium influx triggers the action potential in the afferent nerve ending.

Further reading
1. Ward JP. Oxygen sensors in context. *Biochim Biophys Acta* 2008; 1777 (1): 1-14.
2. Ganong WF, Ed. Carotid and aortic bodies. In: *Review of medical physiology*, 22nd ed. New York, USA: McGraw-Hill, 2005; Chapter 36: 672-5.

2   Answer: D. Proximal tubule in the medulla.

40-50% of filtered urea is reabsorbed through passive diffusion in the proximal convoluted tubules. The Loop of Henle, distal convoluted tubules and cortical collecting ducts are impermeable to urea, but secretion of urea occurs in the descending loop of Henle. This helps to maintain the osmotic gradient in the medulla of the kidney. There is also re-absorption of urea in the medullary collecting ducts.

Further reading
1. Ganong WF, Ed. Water excretion. In: *Review of medical physiology*, 22nd ed. New York, USA: McGraw-Hill, 2005; Chapter 38: 712-20.

3   Answer: B. Passive flow of the blood from atrium to ventricle.

Normally, both atria contract at the same time. Electrical systole is the electrical activity that stimulates the chambers of the heart to make them contract. This is soon followed by mechanical systole, which is the contraction of the heart.

As the atria contract, the pressure in each atrium increases, forcing additional blood into the ventricles. 80% of the blood flows passively down to the ventricles, so the atria do not have to contract a great amount. The remaining filling of the ventricle is due to atrial contraction, which is absent if there is loss of normal electrical conduction in the heart, such as in atrial fibrillation.

Further reading
1. Ganong WF, Ed. Mechanical events of the cardiac cycle. In: *Review of medical physiology*, 22nd ed. New York, USA: McGraw-Hill, 2005; Chapter 29: 565-70.

4   Answer: B. Parathyroid hormone.

Calcium is the most abundant mineral in the human body. The average adult body contains approximately 1kg of calcium in total, 99% in the skeleton in the form of calcium phosphate salts. The serum level of calcium is closely regulated with a normal total calcium of 2.2-2.6mmol/L and a normal ionized calcium of 1.1-1.4mmol/L. The amount of total calcium varies with the level of serum albumin, to which calcium is bound. The biologic effect of calcium is determined by the amount of ionised calcium, rather than the total calcium. Ionised calcium does not vary with the albumin level, and therefore it is useful to measure the ionized calcium level when the serum albumin is not within normal ranges, or when a calcium disorder is suspected despite a normal total calcium level. Primarily, calcium is regulated by the actions of parathyroid hormone (PTH), active vitamin D, calcitonin and direct exchange with the bone matrix. PTH is a very potent regulator of plasma calcium, and controls the conversion of vitamin D into its active form in the kidney. The parafollicular cells of the thyroid produce calcitonin in response to high calcium levels, but its significance is much smaller than that of PTH.

Further reading
1. Ganong WF, Ed. The parathyroid glands. In: *Review of medical physiology*, 22nd ed. New York, USA: McGraw-Hill, 2005; Chapter 21: 390-3.

5   Answer: B. Concentration of protein is very low as compared to that in plasma.

Cerebrospinal fluid (CSF) is considered as a part of the transcellular fluids. The total volume of CSF is 150ml. The daily production is 550ml/day, so CSF turns over about 3 to 4 times per day. The CSF is formed by the choroid plexus (50%) and directly from the walls of the ventricles (50%). CSF flows through the foramens of Magendie and Luschka into the subarachnoid space of the brain and spinal cord. It is absorbed by the arachnoid villi (90%) and directly into cerebral venules (10%). The normal intracerebral pressure (ICP) is 5 to 15mmHg. The rate of formation of CSF is constant and is not affected by ICP. CSF has a composition identical to that of brain ECF but this is different from plasma. The major differences from plasma are: the PCO_2 is higher (50mmHg), resulting in a lower CSF pH (7.33), the protein content is normally very low (0.2g/L) resulting in a low buffering capacity, the glucose concentration is lower, the chloride concentration is higher, and the cholesterol content is very low.

Further reading
1. Johnston M, Papaiconomo C. Cerebrospinal fluid transport: a lymphatic perspective. *Physiological Sciences* 2002; 17: 227-30.

6 Answer: B. Oral metronidazole.

Clostridium difficile infection is associated with broad-spectrum antibiotic therapy and is the most common cause of infectious diarrhoea in hospital patients. Pathogenic strains of *Clostridium difficile* produce exotoxins which cause colonic mucosal injury and inflammation. Infection may be asymptomatic, cause mild diarrhoea, or result in severe pseudomembranous colitis. Diagnosis depends on the demonstration of *Clostridium difficile* toxins in the stool.

The first step in management is to discontinue the antibiotic that caused diarrhoea. If diarrhoea and colitis are severe or persistent, oral metronidazole is the treatment of choice.

Oral vancomycin is also effective, but it is more expensive than metronidazole and its widespread use may encourage the proliferation of vancomycin-resistant nosocomial bacteria.

IV metronidazole may be appropriate for cases of pseudomembranous colitis. Diarrhoea and colitis usually improve within 3 days of commencing metronidazole or vancomycin, but 20% suffer a relapse of diarrhoea when these agents are discontinued. Clarithromycin is not used for the management of *Clostridium difficile* diarrhoea.

Teicoplanin has been used for the treatment of *Clostridium difficile* diarrhoea and there is evidence to suggest that it is better than vancomycin with respect to bacteriologic and symptomatic cure. However, glycopeptide antibiotics such as teicoplanin and vancomycin are reserved for patients who cannot tolerate metronidazole or who do not respond to treatment with it.

Further reading
1. Yentis SM, Hirsch NP, Smith GB. *Anaesthesia and intensive care. A-Z An Encyclopedia of principles and practice*, 3rd ed. Philadelphia, USA: Elsevier, 2005: 123.
2. Kollef MH, Ward S, Sherman G, *et al.* Inadequate treatment of nosocomial infections is associated with certain empiric antibiotic choices. *Critical Care Medicine* 2000; 28: 3456-64.

7 Answer: C. Propofol infusion.

The most likely cause for urine discolouration is medications and food additives. Propofol is metabolized in the liver and excreted in urine predominantly as the 1-glucuronide, 4-glucuronide, and 4-sulfate conjugates of 2,6-diisopropyl-1,4 quinol. Green discolouration of urine is attributed to the presence of these phenolic metabolites. In addition to urine, reports of green discolouration of the hair and liver after propofol administration implicate these phenols.

Atracurium and its metabolites do not cause any urine discolouration. Rifampicin causes a reddish discolouration of the urine. *Klebsiella* and *Pseudomonas* infection may cause colour changes in the urine, but is more commonly observed with urinary tract sepsis than chest infection. Amitryptilline, triamterene, methocarbamol and methylene blue may also cause greenish urine discolouration. Metronidazole, sulphonamides and ferrous salts can cause a brownish discolouration of urine.

Further reading
1. Peck TE, Hill SA, Williams W. Intravenous anaesthetic agents. In: *Pharmacology for anaesthesia and intensive care*, 3rd ed. Cambridge, UK: Cambridge University Press, 2008; Chapter 8: 102-14.
2. Callander CC, Thomas JS, Evans CJ. Propofol and the colour green [letter]. *Anaesthesia* 1989; 44(1): 82.
3. Motsch J, Schmidt H, Bach A, *et al.* Long-term sedation with propofol and green discolouration of the liver. *European Journal of Anaesthesia* 1994; 11: 499-502.

8   Answer: B. Oral fluids and paracetamol.

The history is highly suggestive of postdural puncture headache. She needs to be encouraged to have oral fluids (IV fluids if oral fluids are not tolerated) and simple analgesics (paracetamol) need to be prescribed. If unresponsive, opioids may be prescribed. Caffeine would help by causing vasoconstriction. However, a therapeutic dose may cause atrial fibrillation. Some case series show that desmopressin may be useful in diagnosing and relieving headache. Synthetic ACTH may also be used, but does not have strong enough evidence for regular prescriptions. Desmopressin and caffeine should be avoided in patients with cardiac disease. An epidural blood patch is usually performed for postdural puncture headaches which are unresponsive to conservative management after 24 to 48 hours. If an epidural blood patch is attempted at less than 24 hours after the dural puncture, the success rate is reported to be as low as 29%.

Further reading
1. Harries S, Sivasankar R, *et al*. Postpartum review and problems. In: *Obstetric anaesthesia*, 1st ed. Collis R, Davies S, *et al*. Oxford, UK: Oxford University Press, 2008; Chapter 9: 408-9.
2. Turnbull DK, Shepherd DB. Post-dural puncture headache: pathogenesis, prevention and treatment. *British Journal of Anaesthesia* 2003; 91: 718-29.

9   Answer: D. Repeat adenosine 12mg IV.

Treatment of supraventricular tachycardia in the absence of adverse features includes vagal manoeuvres, followed by adenosine 6mg. In the absence of a satisfactory response, adenosine may be repeated as a 12mg bolus followed by another 12mg.

Since this patient is haemodynamically stable, he does not need electrical cardioversion. Verapamil and adenosine are both effective treatments of supraventricular tachycardia, although some studies have shown that adenosine has a higher success rate and is safer, but transient symptoms are common and arrhythmias may recur.

A common error is to administer intravenous verapamil to a patient with ventricular tachycardia, misdiagnosed as supraventricular tachycardia. In this setting, hypotension and ventricular fibrillation can occur.

Verapamil can induce atrioventricular block when used in large doses or in patients with atrioventricular nodal disease.

Further reading
1. http://www.resus.org.uk/pages/periarst.pdf.
2. Ferguson JD, DiMarco JP. Contemporary management of paroxysmal supraventricular tachycardia. *Circulation* 2003; 107: 1096-9.

10 Answer: B. 3mg of morphine.

Morphine is a weak base, therefore, it is ionised in the acidic gastric environment. This would delay its absorption until it reaches the alkaline environment of the small bowel where it becomes unionised. Peak levels after oral administration are much lower than after parenteral routes, since it undergoes extensive first pass metabolism and only approximately 30% reaches the systemic circulation. With repeated administration, the oral-parenteral relative potency ratio is 1:3. With therapeutic doses, plasma protein binding is only 20-35%, and the volume of distribution is 1-6L/kg. The primary site of morphine metabolism is the liver, and the dose should be reduced in patients with liver disease. Glucuronidation is the main metabolic pathway, but the principal metabolite, morphine-3-glucuronide (M3G), is inactive. Morphine-6-glucuronide (M6G) is produced in smaller amounts than M3G, but is pharmacologically active and many times more potent than morphine.

Further reading
1. Peck TE, Hill SA, Williams M, Eds. Opioid-related drugs. In: *Pharmacology for anaesthesia and intensive care*, 3rd ed. Cambridge, UK: Cambridge University Press 2008; Chapter 9: 135-49.

11   Answer: E. Hypoventilation.

This patient is breathing spontaneously through a laryngeal mask airway. In an elderly patient, 1.5 MAC of isoflurane along with intermittent boluses of fentanyl is likely to result in hypoventilation. This is further supported by low oxygen saturation.

Malignant hyperthermia is characterised by an unexplained rise in $EtCO_2$, tachycardia, hyperthermia, acidosis and muscle rigidity. Malfunction of inspiratory and expiratory unidirectional valves and exhausted sodalime will result in rebreathing of exhaled CO_2. In this case, the clinical scenario is suggestive of increased depth of anaesthesia. The management involves checking the other vital parameters, such as blood pressure, heart rate and respiratory rate and reducing the depth of anaesthesia. Meanwhile, other causes of hypercapnia should be excluded.

Further reading
1. Al-Shaikh B, Stacey S. Sodalime and circle breathing system. *Essentials of anaesthetic equipment*, 3rd ed. London, UK: Churchill Livingstone, Elsevier, 2007; 4: 56-8.
2. Laffey JG, Kavanagh BP. Hypocapnia. *New England Journal of Medicine* 2002; 347: 43-53.

12   Answer: D. Vigilant anaesthetist continuously monitoring chest wall excursion.

Monitoring devices supplement clinical observation. A vigilant anaesthetist is the vital link interpreting the monitoring and acting immediately to appropriately manage the critical incident. There are several disconnection monitors used in clinical practice. However, the most important monitor is a vigilant anaesthetist who can interpret the physiological and mechanical (spirometry and pressure sensor) monitors. Disconnection of the breathing system can be detected using the following measures.

- Clinical observation:
   - chest wall excursion;
   - movement of ventilator bellows;
   - absence of breath sounds.

◆ Mechanical monitors:
  - pneumotachograph;
  - pressure sensors;
  - capnography.

Monitoring $EtCO_2$ is probably the best monitor in revealing patient disconnections. However, there may still be an $EtCO_2$ reading with a partial disconnection. Similarly, the absence of $EtCO_2$ due to circulatory arrest or a low reading due to a small leak in the sampling line can be mistaken for a disconnection of the breathing system.

Further reading
1. Recommendations for standards of monitoring during anaesthesia and recovery, 4th ed. Association of Anaesthetists of Great Britain and Ireland, 2007. http://www.aagbi.org/publications/guidelines/docs/standardsofmonitoring07.pdf.
2. Brockwell RC, Andrews JJ. Inhaled anesthetic delivery systems. In: *Miller's anesthesia*, Volume 1, 7th ed. Miller RD, Ed. Philadelphia, USA: Churchill Livingstone, 2010; Chapter 25: 667-710.

13 Answer: B. Transoesophageal echocardiography.

Venous air embolism (VAE) is a recognised complication of surgery in the sitting position, in posterior fossa surgery and in head and neck surgery in a head-up position. The factors facilitating air entrainment include open veins, negative intravenous pressure relative to atmospheric pressure and low central venous pressure due to the gravity effect.

The monitoring techniques in order of decreasing sensitivity include: transoesophageal echocardiography, precordial Doppler, pulmonary artery pressure measurement, end-tidal CO_2 monitoring, right atrial pressure measurement and oesophageal stethoscope.

During posterior fossa surgery in the sitting position, VAE has been detectable by precordial Doppler in approximately 40% of patients and by transoesophageal echocardiography in 76% of patients. The incidence of VAE is much less during posterior fossa surgery in the non-sitting position. There is also a risk of paradoxical air embolism through a patent foramen ovale. The management of VAE involves lowering the head, flooding the surgical field with saline, aspirating air through the central venous catheter and cardiovascular support.

Further reading
1. Porter JM, Pidgeon C, Cunningham AJ. The sitting position in neurosurgery: a critical appraisal. *British Journal of Anaesthesia* 1999; 82: 117-28.
2. Drummond JC, Patel PM. Neurosurgical anesthesia. In: *Miller's anesthesia*, Volume 1, 7th ed. Miller RD, Ed. Philadelphia, USA: Churchill Livingstone, 2010; Chapter 63: 2045-87.
3. Fathi A-R, Eshtehardi P, Meier B. Patent foramen ovale and neurosurgery in sitting position: a systematic review. *British Journal of Anaesthesia* 2009; 102(5): 588-96.

14 Answer: B. Monitoring inspired oxygen concentration very close to the endotracheal tube.

In a completely closed system all the exhaled gases are rebreathed except for CO_2 which is absorbed by the sodalime or baralime. The oxygen concentration in the exhaled gas mixture depends on the inspired oxygen concentration and alveolar oxygen extraction. The initial concentration of oxygen measured at the common gas outlet and anaesthetic agent concentration (dial setting) in the fresh gas flow are diluted in the circle system. The oxygen concentration gradually decreases over time due to the dilution effect from exhaled gases in the circle system. Therefore, it is essential to monitor the inspired oxygen concentration close to the endotracheal tube. Paramagnetic type oxygen analysers allow breath-to-breath measurement of oxygen concentration.

Monitoring of inspired CO_2 concentration is useful in detecting an exhausted CO_2 absorber (sodalime).

Further reading
1. Davey AJ. Breathing systems and their components. In: *Ward's anaesthetic equipment*, 5th ed. Davey AJ, Diba A, Eds. Philadelphia, USA: Elsevier Saunders, 2005; Chapter 7: 131-63.

15 Answer: A. One.

The pressure in the full oxygen cylinder is 137 bar and the volume of the cylinder is 5L. A full size E oxygen cylinder contains 685L (137 x 5) of oxygen. But 5L will remain in the cylinder, so the available volume is 680L. Since the ventilator requires 20 bar of pressure to operate, it will stop operating when the cylinder pressure reaches 20 bar. Therefore, the available oxygen for clinical use is 580L (117 x 5 = 585-5). The total oxygen consumption is 10L per minute (5L is for ventilating the patient's lungs and 5L for driving the ventilator). So the cylinder should last for 58 minutes. Therefore, one full cylinder of oxygen is required for the journey. However, in practical terms, one should ensure that double the amount of calculated oxygen is available to overcome any delays that may arise during transfer.

Further reading
1. Davis PD, Kenny GNC. The gas laws. In: *Basic physics and measurement in anaesthesia*, 5th ed. London, UK: Butterworth-Heinemann, 2003: 37-50.
2. Bland H. The supply of anaesthetic and other medical gases. In: Davey AJ, Diba Ali, Eds. *Ward's anaesthetic equipment*, 5th ed. Philadelphia, USA: Elsevier Saunders, 2005: 23-49.

16 Answer: E. Helium.

Nitrogen narcosis while diving is a reversible alteration in consciousness that occurs while scuba diving at depth. Narcosis produces a state similar to alcohol intoxication or nitrous oxide inhalation, and can occur during shallow dives, but it is not usually noticeable until depths beyond 30m (100ft).

Apart from helium, and probably neon, all gases that can be breathed have a narcotic effect, which is greater as the lipid solubility of the gas increases. The condition is completely reversed by ascending to a shallower depth with no long-term effects. Diving beyond 40m (130ft) is considered outside the scope of recreational diving as narcosis and oxygen toxicity become critical factors, and specialist training is required in the use of various gas mixtures such as heliox.

Further reading
1. Bennett P, Rostain JC. Inert gas narcosis. In: *Bennett and Elliott's physiology and medicine of diving*, 5th ed. Brubakk AO, Neuman TS, Eds. USA: Saunders Ltd, 2003: 304.

17 Answer: A. Zone 1.

The hepatic acinus is the functional unit of the liver. The acinus represents a unit that is of more relevance to hepatic function because it is oriented around the afferent vascular system. The acinus consists of an irregular-shaped, roughly ellipsoidal mass of hepatocytes aligned around the hepatic arterioles and portal venules just as they anastomose into sinusoids. The acinus is roughly divided into zones that correspond to distance from the arterial blood supply (Figure 1): those hepatocytes closest to the arterioles (zone 1 below) are the best oxygenated, while those farthest from the arterioles have the poorest supply of oxygen. This arrangement also means that cells in the center of the acinus (again, zone 1) are the first to be exposed to blood-borne toxins absorbed into portal blood from the small intestine. The net result is that a variety of pathologic processes lead to lesions that reflect acinar structure.

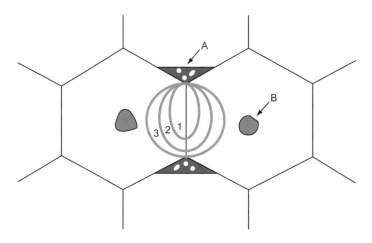

Figure 1. Structure of hepatic acinus. A = portal space containing the bile duct, portal vein and hepatic artery. B = central vein. 1, 2 and 3 represent zones 1, 2 and 3.

Further reading
1. Ganong WF, Ed. Liver & biliary system. In: *Review of medical physiology*, 22nd ed. New York, USA: McGraw-Hill, 2005; Chapter 26: 498-504.

18 Answer: D. Evaporation.

There are four mechanisms of heat loss: convection, conduction, radiation, and evaporation. If body temperature is greater than that of the surroundings, the body can lose heat by radiation and conduction. But if the temperature of the surroundings is greater than that of the skin, the body actually gains heat by radiation and conduction. In such conditions, the only means by which the body can rid itself of heat is by evaporation. During sports activities, evaporation becomes the main avenue of heat loss. Humidity affects thermoregulation by limiting sweat evaporation and thus heat loss.

Further reading
1. Ganong WF, Ed. Temperature regulation. In: *Review of medical physiology*, 22nd cd. New York, USA: McGraw-Hill, 2005; Chapter 14: 251-5.

19 Answer: B. Partial pressure of CO_2.

Cerebral blood flow (CBF) in an adult is 750ml/minute or 15% of the cardiac output. This equates to 50ml of blood/100g of brain tissue/minute. CBF is tightly regulated to meet the brain's metabolic demands. Cerebral blood flow is determined by a number of factors, such as viscosity of blood, vasodilatation or vasoconstriction of cerebral vessels and cerebral perfusion pressure (CPP). The CPP is dependent on the difference between the mean blood pressure and intracranial pressure. CBF is autoregulated. Cerebral arterioles constrict and dilate in response to different chemical concentrations. For example, they dilate in response to higher levels of CO_2 or lower levels of oxygen. Carbon dioxide is a potent vasodilator of cerebral blood vessels and the slightest change in PCO_2 affects the CBF.

Changes in intracranial pressure, blood pressure, temperature, and partial pressure of oxygen need to be significant, when compared to PCO_2, to affect CBF.

Further reading
1. Kandel ER, Schwartz JH, Jessell TM. *Principles of neural science*, 4th ed. New York, USA: McGraw-Hill, 2000: 1305.

20 Answer: D. Sustained increase in the secretion of hormones in the posterior pituitary gland.

Chronically increased blood pressure can be caused by a sustained increase in the secretion of hormones of the adrenal medulla such as aldosterone and glucocorticoids. Long-term treatment with oral contraceptives which contain oestrogens can cause significant hypertension in some women. This is due to an oestrogen-induced increase in circulating levels of angiotensinogen.

The hormones secreted by the posterior pituitary have no role in regulation of blood pressure and, therefore, a sustained increase in their secretion does not cause hypertension.

Further reading
1. Ganong WF, Ed. Hypertension in humans. In: *Review of medical physiology,* 22nd ed. New York, USA: McGraw-Hill, 2005; Chapter 33: 641-2.

21 Answer: B. Pulmonary function tests.

Patients with severe rheumatoid arthritis can have restrictive lung disease. This patient is also on methotrexate, amiodarone and leflunamide - all these drugs can cause pulmonary fibrosis. Pulmonary function testing would be the most appropriate special investigation of all the investigations mentioned. An echocardiogram would give information about the patient's left ventricular function, and presence of a thrombus in the atrium. A transoesophageal echocardiogram (TOE) is not indicated as a first-line investigation. TOE may be considered if a transthoracic echocardiogram does not provide good images.

Polymyalgia rheumatica (PMR) is a chronic, episodic, inflammatory disease of the large arteries that usually develops in people over 50 years of age. The diagnosis is generally based on the clinical syndrome, an elevated ESR and a response to a therapeutic trial of a low-dose steroid. An electromyogram or muscle biopsy is not indicated in confirming the diagnosis. Although a coagulation screen is usually performed as a routine investigation, there is no absolute indication in this patient.

Other investigations that should be performed in this patient are a 12-lead ECG, and serum electrolytes. A 12-lead electrocardiogram is important, as it would give information about the rate, rhythm, axis and ST segment changes. Measurement of blood urea, serum creatinine and electrolytes are indicated in an elderly patient. In this patient any abnormal electrolytes, particularly serum potassium, should be corrected.

Further reading
1. Fombon FN, Thompson JP. Anaesthesia for the adult patient with rheumatoid arthritis. *British Journal of Anaesthesia CEACCP* 2006; 6: 235-9.

22 Answer: A. Leave arterial line *in situ*, inject procaine and perform a stellate ganglion block.

Following intra-arterial injection of thiopentone, the cannula is preferably left *in situ* as the artery would be in severe spasm. Heparin, procaine (for analgesia), papaverine or tolazoline (for vasodilatation) may be injected into the artery. A sympathetic block should be performed to overcome vasospasm - either a stellate ganglion block or brachial plexus block. Although administration of intravenous heparin is likely to reduce the arterial thrombosis, it should be withheld until the stellate ganglion block has been performed to reduce the risk of bleeding.

Further reading
1. Yentis SM, Hirsch NP, Smith GB. *Anaesthesia and intensive care. A-Z An encyclopedia of principles and practice*, 3rd ed. Philadelphia, USA: Elsevier, 2005: 507-8.

23 Answer: B. Erythromycin.

Gastrointestinal promotility agents increase contractile force and accelerate intraluminal transit. They may improve tolerance to enteral nutrition, reduce gastroesophageal reflux and pulmonary aspiration and, therefore, have the potential to improve outcomes of critically ill patients. Erythromycin is a macrolide antibiotic, which at low doses acts as a prokinetic drug. Erythromycin involves two different pathways and its effects are dose-dependent. It acts on motilin receptors, which are present on enteric nerves and smooth muscle, to increase antral activity with caudal migration of peristaltic waves. It also activates the intrinsic cholinergic pathway.

At a low dose (40mg), it induces premature activity at the antral level, migrating caudally to the small intestine. This may be mediated by the activation of an intrinsic cholinergic pathway. At higher doses (200-350mg), it induces a prolonged period of strong antral activity without any peristaltic activity, which is possibly mediated via a pathway that involves the activation of motilin. The other drugs - ondansetron, prochlorperazine, dexamethasone, cyclizine - do not have any prokinetic action. They are used as anti-emetic drugs. Metoclopramide and cisapride are other prokinetic agents, which have been used in critical care for the purposes of enteric tube placement and enteral feeding.

Further reading
1. Booth CM, Heyland DK, Paterson WG. Gastrointestinal promotility drugs in the critical care setting: a systematic review of the evidence. *Critical Care Medicine* 2002; 30: 1429-35.

24 Answer: C. Intramuscular oxytocin and ergometrine.

Oxytocin acts directly on the receptors on the uterine myometrium, increasing the force and frequency of contractions. It is administered intravenously as a bolus dose of 5mg followed by an intravenous infusion if required. A bolus dose of >5U can produce tachycardia and hypotension due to reduced systemic vascular resistance.

Ergometrine is usually administered intramuscularly together with oxytocin (Syntometrine® contains 5U of Syntocinon® and 500g of ergometrine). Syntometrine® combines the rapid action of Syntocinon® with the sustained uterotonic effect of ergometrine.

20U of oxytocin, if administered as an intravenous bolus, would result in significant haemodynamic effects.

Salbutamol is a tocolytic and is contraindicated at this stage. It acts on the two receptors on the uterus and causes smooth muscle relaxation. This would further relax the uterus and may cause postpartum haemorrhage.

Prostaglandin F or E may be used but they should not be given intravenously for uterine contraction at this stage. Intravenous prostaglandin has been used for the purposes of induction of labour. Misoprostol (prostaglandin E1) is given PR, and is no longer administered as an intramyometrial injection.

Further reading
1. Eggers K, Chawathe M, *et al.* Drugs for uterine contraction. In: *Obstetric anaesthesia*, 1st ed, Collis R, Davies S, *et al.* Oxford, UK: Oxford University Press, 2008; Chapter 9: 278-80.

25 Answer: A. Hyperkalaemia.

Hyperkalaemia is common in patients with renal impairment. Angiotensin-converting enzyme inhibitors (ACE-I) (enalapril) and potassium-sparing diuretics (spironolactone) further predispose to hyperkalaemia.

This patient may also be susceptible to hyponatraemia due to reduced aldosterone secretion. Spironolactone, a potassium-sparing diuretic, is a synthetic steroid that acts as a competitive antagonist to aldosterone. Hypokalaemia eventually develops in many patients who are on loop diuretics or thiazides. This can usually be managed with dietary restriction of sodium chloride or with dietary potassium supplements. If hypokalaemia persists, then the addition of a potassium-sparing diuretic can help in correcting hypokalaemia by reducing K^+ excretion. Although this approach is generally safe, it should be avoided in patients with renal insufficiency and in those receiving angiotensin antagonists such as ACE-Is, as life-threatening hyperkalaemia can develop in response to potassium-sparing diuretics.

Hypocalcaemia would not be caused by any of the drugs being taken by this patient. Spironolactone in combination with ACE-Is may alter the serum magnesium levels, although this is not a consistent effect. The chronic use of loop diuretics may cause hypomagnesaemia.

Further reading
1. Peck TE, Hill SA, Williams M, Eds. Diuretics. In: *Pharmacology for anaesthesia and intensive care*, 3rd ed. Cambridge, UK: Cambridge University Press, 2008; Chapter 21: 305-10.

26 Answer: E. 77.6mmHg.

The transducer system is zeroed with the reference point of the transducer at the level of the aortic root to eliminate the effect of the fluid column of the system on blood pressure readings. Once zeroed, the transducer should be maintained at the same reference point. Since the table is lowered by 10cm, the transducer is now 10cm higher than the original reference point. Therefore, it underestimates blood pressure by 10cm H_2O which is equivalent to 7.6mmHg.

Further reading
1. Bedford RF, Shah NK. Blood pressure monitoring. In: *Monitoring in anaesthesia and critical care*, 3rd ed. Blitt CD, Hines RL, Eds. New York, USA: Churchill Livingstone, 1995: 95-130.

27 Answer: A. Dental trauma.

The most frequent complication associated with direct laryngscopy and tracheal intubation is dental trauma. Should dental trauma occur, one should immediately consult a dentist for further advice. Although claims related to dental damage are numerically high, financially they contribute to a proportionally low total claim.

Further reading
1. Cook TM, Scott S, Mihai R. Litigation-related airway and respiratory complications of anaesthesia: an analysis of claims against the NHS in England 1995-2007. *Anaesthesia* 2010; 65: 556-63.

28 Answer: D. Reflection of ultrasound beam at tissue interfaces.

Ultrasound is now widely used in anaesthetic practice for imaging neurovascular structures and for diagnostic and therapeutic imaging in intensive care. The characteristics of an ultrasound beam are described in terms of frequency, wavelength and amplitude.

A low frequency ultrasound beam has a longer wavelength and greater penetration of deeper tissues, but poorer image resolution. For example, frequencies of 3-5MHz are used for abdominal scanning, whereas for imaging superficial structures in the neck, frequencies in the range of 10-12MHz are used.

When the ultrasound waves reach the tissue boundary (at the junction of two tissue planes of different density), part of the ultrasound is reflected and part of the wave is transmitted. The magnitude of the reflected beam depends on the difference between the two impedances. The impedance depends on the speed of ultrasound in the tissue and density of the tissue. As the same transducer is used to transmit and receive the ultrasound waves, the time taken for the ultrasound wave to travel and return enables measurement of the depth of boundary from the surface.

Further reading
1. Ultrasound. In: *Principles of measurement and monitoring in anaesthesia and intensive care*, 3rd ed. Sykes MK, Vickers MD, Hull CJ, Eds. Oxford, UK: Blackwell Scientific Publications, 1991; Chapter 9: 160-17.
2. Marhofer P, Ed. Basic principles of ultrasonography. In: *Ultrasound guidance in regional anaesthesia, principles and practical implementation.* Oxford, UK: Oxford University Press, 2010; Chapter 1: 1-19.

29   Answer: E. Three twitches on TOF response.

Depth of neuromuscular blockade can be measured using several modes of stimulation such as single twitch, train-of-four, double-burst stimulation, tetanic stimulation and post-tetanic count. Train-of-four is more commonly used both during maintenance and recovery of anaesthesia. It involves stimulating the nerve with four supra-maximal twitch stimuli with a frequency of 2Hz. TOF can be repeated every 10 seconds. If non-depolarizing blockade is present, there will be a loss of twitch height and number, which will indicate the degree of blockade. The presence of no twitches in the TOF response indicates deep muscle blockade and is ideal for intubation. At least three twitches should be present prior to administration of reversal agent. To ensure satisfactory recovery from neuromuscular blockade, the TOF ratio should be >0.9 at extubation.

Further reading

1. Ali HH, Savarese JJ, *et al*. Twitch, tetanus and train-of-four as indices of recovery from nondepolarizing neuromuscular blockade. *Anaesthesiology* 2003; 98(5): 1278-80.
2. McGrath CD, Hunter JF. Monitoring of neuromuscular block. *British Journal of Anaesthesia CEACCP* 2006; 6: 7-12.

30   Answer: E. The dilutional effect of rebreathing.

This is a common clinical observation during low-flow anaesthesia. The dilutional effect of rebreathing contributes to the difference between the dial setting and inspired concentration. The dial setting on the vaporiser reflects the concentration delivered to the breathing system. The inspired concentration detected by the agent analyser reflects the concentration of anaesthetic agent at the tracheal tube end of the breathing system.

In low-flow anaesthesia, exhaled gases are recirculated after eliminating the CO_2 through the CO_2 absorber (sodalime or baralime). The minute volume is composed of the fresh gas flow (FGF) and the recirculated and rebreathed exhaled gases. As FGF is decreased, the exhaled patient gases contribute a more significant portion of the minute volume. In this scenario, anaesthesia is maintained with a low FGF of 0.3L/minute; the most likely reason for the difference is a dilution effect of the rebreathed gases.

Malfunction of the vaporiser can deliver a lower concentration of anesthetic and malfunction of the agent analyser can also account for the inaccuracy in the measured concentration. Increased uptake of volatile agent by the patient accounts for the increased difference between the inspired and expired concentration rather than increased difference between the dial setting and inspired concentration.

Further reading
1. Hendrickx JFA, Coddens J, Callebaut F, *et al*. Effect of N_2O on sevoflurane vaporizer settings during minimal- and low-flow anesthesia. *Anesthesiology* 2002; 97: 400-4.
2. Philiph JH. The dilution effect of rebreathing. www.gehealthcare.com/usen/anesthesia/docs/DilutionEffect.

Set 6 questions

1   A 36-year-old primigravida, with a history of polyhydramnios delivers a baby at 34 weeks' gestation. The midwife notices that the baby chokes and persistently coughs on attempted feeding. Which of the following anatomical tracheo-oesophageal fistulae is most likely to be the cause for these symptoms in the neonate?

a.   The upper segment ends as a blind pouch and the lower segment communicates with the trachea.

b.   The upper segment communicates with the trachea and the lower segment ends as a blind pouch.

c.   Both upper and lower segments end as blind pouches.

d.   The upper segment communicates with the lower part of the trachea and the lower segment arises from the carina.

e.   The two segments join together and communicate with the lower part of the trachea.

2   A 60-year-old female patient underwent a laparotomy with extensive small bowel resection. She has now developed an entero-cutaneous fistula. As a result she is on parenteral nutrition via a central venous catheter inserted through the internal jugular vein. Which of the following complications is most likely in this patient?

a.   Venous thrombosis.

b.   Symptomatic liver disease.

c.   Osteoporosis.

d.   Osteomalacia.

e.   Catheter infection.

3   You are performing spinal anaesthesia on a 65-year-old male patient in the right lateral position for an inguinal hernia repair. As you advance the spinal needle, he complains of sharp stabbing pain in his right leg. The next most appropriate step in the management is:

a.   Abandon the procedure.
b.   Advance the needle further inwards in the same direction.
c.   Withdraw the needle and redirect more medially.
d.   Withdraw the needle and direct laterally.
e.   Inject more local anaesthetic.

4   During exercise, blood flow to muscles increases significantly. Which one of the following is most likely to contribute to the initial rise in skeletal muscle blood flow at the beginning of exercise?

a.   Vasodilatation of blood vessels due to local metabolites.
b.   Increased sympathetic discharge to peripheral vessels.
c.   Increase in cardiac output.
d.   Increase in arterial blood pressure.
e.   Increase in heart rate.

5   You have administered 2L of colloid solution to an anaesthetised 43-year-old healthy male. Which one of the following blood vessels will best accommodate the change in circulatory volume?

a.   Systemic arteries.
b.   Systemic veins.
c.   Systemic capillaries.
d.   Pulmonary capillaries.
e.   Pulmonary veins.

6   A 20-year-old male patient is scheduled for an emergency appendicectomy. There is a family history of suxamethonium apnoea. When he was investigated for suxamethonium apnoea, blood tests revealed a dibucaine number of 20 and a genotype of Ea: Ea

(homozygous atypical). Which of the following muscle relaxants is most suitable for rapid sequence induction in this patient?

a.   Suxamethonium 1mg/kg.
b.   Rocuronium 0.9mg/kg.
c.   Rocuronium 0.3mg/kg.
d.   Rocuronium 0.6mg/kg.
e.   Rocuronium 0.5mg/kg.

7   A 45-year-old female patient is scheduled for extraction of one pre-molar tooth under local anaesthesia and sedation. She has hypertension which is treated with atenolol 50mg. After establishing baseline monitoring, fentanyl 75µg was administered in aliquots every 2-3 minutes. She also received 0.5mg of midazolam. Subsequently, the surgeon infiltrated 3ml of 3% prilocaine with felypressin. At this stage she required another 50µg of fentanyl intravenously. She became very rigid and complained of difficulty in breathing with tightness in her chest. Which of the following drugs is the most likely cause for this?

a.   Midazolam.
b.   Felypressin.
c.   Prilocaine.
d.   Fentanyl.
e.   Atenolol.

8   Inhalational anaesthetic agents affect systemic vascular resistance (SVR). Which one of the following agents has the least effect on SVR?

a.   Isoflurane.
b.   Sevoflurane.
c.   Desflurane.
d.   Enflurane.
e.   Halothane.

9 Protein binding of a local anaesthetic determines its duration of action. Which one of the following sequences correctly indicates the level of protein binding of local anaesthetics in a decreasing order?

a. Procaine > bupivacaine > lignocaine > prilocaine.
b. Bupivacaine > lignocaine > prilocaine > procaine.
c. Prilocaine > bupivacaine > lignocaine > prilocaine.
d. Lignocaine > bupivacaine > prilocaine > procaine.
e. Bupivacaine > lignocaine > procaine > prilocaine.

10 Which one of the following mechanisms best explains the reason for using sodium nitrite in the management of cyanide toxicity?

a. It increases methaemoglobinaemia.
b. It produces increased hepatic sulphydryl groups.
c. It increases the conversion to cyanocobalamin.
d. It displaces cyanide from haemoglobin.
e. It enhances oxidative phosphorylation.

11 The graph below describes the relationship between true blood pressure and measured blood pressure through an invasive arterial cannula connected to a transducer system (Figure 1). Line A represents the ideal response. Lines B and C represent false readings due to a calibration error. The error represented by line C can best be corrected by:

a. Zeroing the system.
b. Replacing the transducer cable.
c. Performing a three-point calibration.
d. Performing a two-point calibration.
e. Performing a square wave test.

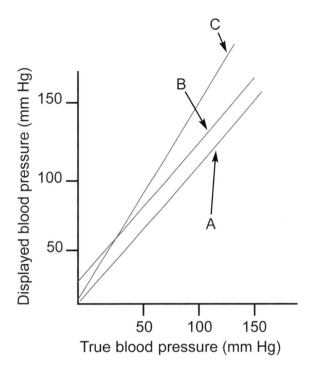

Figure 1. The relationship between true blood pressure and measured blood pressure through an invasive arterial cannula connected to a transducer system.

12 You are planning to perform inhalational induction using sevoflurane on an adult patient weighing 68kg. Which of the following is the most efficient breathing system for this purpose?

a. Mapleson D system.
b. Mapleson A system.
c. Mapleson B system.
d. Mapleson C System.
e. The Bain system.

13 A 45-year-old female presents for a laparoscopic cholecystectomy. General anaesthesia using intravenous induction followed by maintenance with volatile agents is planned. In view of avoiding awareness, which of the following monitors is most useful?

a.	Isolated forearm technique.
b.	Bispectral index.
c.	Minimum alveolar concentration (MAC) of volatile anaesthetic agent.
d.	Lower oesophageal contractility.
e.	Late cortical evoked responses.

14 You are planning to evaluate three fluid warmers in a laboratory setting. You need to accurately monitor the temperature of the fluid and would like to detect a very small difference of up to 0.001°C. Which of the following temperature measurement devices is most suitable for this research?

a.	Mercury thermometer.
b.	Infrared thermometer.
c.	Platinum resistance thermometer.
d.	Thermistor.
e.	Bourdon gauge thermometer.

15 You are planning to undertake research to evaluate the intubating conditions of a new non-depolarising muscle relaxant. Which of the following peripheral muscle and nerve combinations is most appropriate for this purpose?

a.	Ulnar nerve and adductor pollicis.
b.	Facial nerve and orbicularis occuli.
c.	Tibial nerve and abductor hallucis.
d.	Common peroneal nerve (lateral popliteal) and extensor hallucis longus.
e.	Facial nerve and orbicularis oris.

16 Airway resistance varies along different parts of the respiratory tract. In which of the following areas is the airway resistance greatest?

a. Trachea.
b. Terminal bronchioles.
c. Medium-sized bronchi.
d. Alveoli.
e. Alveolar ducts.

17 A 28-year-old male is admitted to the ICU after taking a drug overdose. He is comatose and about to be intubated. His $PaCO_2$ was 5.3kPa ten minutes ago, but you discover it is now 9kPa. Which one of the following statements is most likely to be true about this patient?

a. The pH of his CSF is likely to fall more slowly than the pH of his blood.
b. The pH of his blood is likely to fall more slowly than the pH of his CSF.
c. The pH of his blood and CSF will not change because he will rapidly eliminate bicarbonate in the urine in response to the rise in $PaCO_2$.
d. The pH of his blood will fall immediately without any change in the pH of his CSF.
e. The pH of his blood will fall and the pH of his CSF will rise over the next 24 hours.

18 A patient ingests antifreeze and needs to eliminate the ingested acid. Renal elimination of the protons of this excess acid is primarily accomplished by which of the following mechanisms?

a. Increased urinary ammonium excretion.
b. Increased urinary excretion of phosphates.
c. Hyperventilation.
d. Increased urinary free hydrogen ion concentration.
e. Increased urinary sulfate excretion.

19 A number of conditions affect the structure or concentration of haemoglobin in blood. Which one of the following conditions is most likely to be associated with a reduced level but normal structure of haemoglobin in the blood?

a. Thalassaemia.
b. Anaemia due to chronic blood loss.
c. Blood transfusion reaction.
d. Haemolytic anaemia.
e. Sickle cell anaemia.

20 A 29-year-old female has puffy skin, a hoarse voice and complains of an intolerance to cold. Her plasma thyroid stimulating hormone (TSH) level is low and this increases significantly if she is given thyrotropin releasing hormone (TRH). Which one of the following is the most likely diagnosis in this woman?

a. Hypothyroidism due a primary abnormality in the pituitary gland.
b. Hyperthyroidism due to a thyroid tumour.
c. Hypothyroidism due to a thyroid tumour.
d. Hyperthyroidism due to a primary abnormality in the hypothalamus.
e. Hypothyroidism due to a primary abnormality in the hypothalamus.

21 A 78-year-old male patient with arthritis, hypertension and congestive cardiac failure is scheduled to have an open prostatectomy. He is on bendrofluazide 5mg o.d., and amiloride 20mg o.d. He is seen in the pre-operative assessment clinic and routine blood tests have been ordered. The most likely abnormal biochemical finding in the blood is:

a. Hyponatraemia.
b. Hyperuricaemia.
c. Hyperphosphataemia.
d. Hypomagnesaemia.
e. Hypercalcaemia.

22 A 64-year-old male is listed for excision of a ganglion on the wrist. He suffers from rheumatoid arthritis and asthma. He takes his salbutamol inhaler 200µg t.d.s. and prednisolone 15mg once a day. He has been on these drugs for over 2 years. Which of the following is the most appropriate with regard to his peri-operative management?

a. Prednisolone 15mg on the morning of surgery.
b. Hydrocortisone 100mg at induction.
c. Hydrocortisone 50mg at induction and 50mg 6 hours postoperatively.
d. Prednisolone 15mg on the morning of surgery and hydrocortisone 50mg at induction.
e. Hydrocortisone 100mg at induction and 50mg 6 hours postoperatively.

23 A 62-year-old male patient with end-stage liver disease and cirrhosis is scheduled for an emergency laparotomy. Which of the following non-depolarising neuromuscular blocking agents is most suitable for this patient?

a. Vecuronium.
b. Pancuronium.
c. Mivacurium.
d. Rocuronium.
e. Atracurium.

24 A 46-year-old male is diagnosed with a vascular occlusion in his left leg. He is taken to the emergency theatre for an embolectomy and femoral cross-over graft surgery. He is known to have end-stage renal disease and is on daily peritoneal dialysis. He is in the

anaesthetic room for induction. His ECG shows a prolonged PR interval and tall T waves. His blood results are shown in Table 1.

Table 1. Blood results.			
Na+	K+	Urea	Creatinine
139mmol/L	7.2mmol/L	15mmol/L	182µmol/L

Which of the following is the next immediate step in the management of hyperkalaemia?

a.   Intravenous 10ml of 10% calcium chloride over 5 minutes.
b.   Intravenous salbutamol 250µg.
c.   Intravenous insulin 50 units over an hour.
d.   Intravenous furosemide 20mg.
e.   Intravenous sodium bicarbonate 50mmols over an hour.

25 A 30-year-old male is due to undergo an urgent laparotomy. He has a family history of suxamethonium apnoea. Induction with propofol and rocuronium is planned. In the event of an unanticipated failed intubation, which of the following is the most appropriate in reversing the neuromuscular blockade?

a.   Intravenous neostigmine 0.07mg/kg and glycopyrrolate 0.01mg/kg.
b.   Intravenous neostigmine 0.1mg/kg and glycopyrrolate 0.05mg/kg.
c.   Intravenous sugammadex 16mg/kg.
d.   Intravenous sugammadex 4mg/kg.
e.   Intravenous edrophonium 0.1mg/kg.

26 You are anaesthetising a patient at high altitude where atmospheric pressure is 380mm Hg. If the set concentration on the isoflurane

vaporiser is 2%, in reality which one of the following indicates the correct concentration of vapour delivered in the inspiratory flow to the patient?

a.   1%.
b.   2%.
c.   3%.
d.   4%.
e.   0.5%.

27 A defibrillator has a capacitor with a potential of 4000 Volts and a charge of 0.2 coulombs. What will be the maximum stored energy in this defibrillator?

a.   100J.
b.   150J.
c.   360J.
d.   400J.
e.   460J.

28 A 60-year-old female patient is scheduled to undergo a vaginal hysterectomy in the lithotomy position under general anaesthesia. The anticipated surgical duration is 75 minutes. Which one of the following characteristics of a ProSeal® LMA makes it most suitable over a classic LMA?

a.   Presence of a flexible wire reinforced airway tube.
b.   Better haemodynamic stability as compared to a classic LMA.
c.   Reduced incidence of cough and sore throat in the postoperative period.
d.   Improved airway seal, enabling positive pressure ventilation.
e.   Shorter and reinforced tube with an integral bite block.

29 A 72-year-old male patient is scheduled to undergo a total hip replacement under spinal anaesthesia. You have administered spinal anaesthesia using 2.6ml of 0.5% heavy bupivacaine. Which of the following is least useful in assessing the height of block?

a.   Peripheral oxygen saturation.
b.   Bispectral index monitoring.
c.   Checking the level of touch sensation.
d.   Monitoring blood pressure.
e.   Checking the level of cold sensation.

30 A 68-year-old male patient is undergoing a total knee replacement. The airway is secured with an i-Gel® supraglottic airway. Anaesthesia is maintained with sevoflurane 2.5% in oxygen and nitrous oxide with a total fresh gas flow of 0.8L/minute through a circle breathing system. The patient is breathing spontaneously. About an hour after starting the procedure, the patient showed signs of being in a light plane of anaesthesia, despite the sevoflurane dial set at 3%. The inspired sevoflurane is 2.6% and expired sevoflurane is 1.2%. Which of the following is the most likely cause for the gross difference in the inspired and expired concentration of sevoflurane?

a.   Malfunction of the vaporiser.
b.   Malfunction of the vapour analyser.
c.   Increased uptake of sevoflurane by the patient.
d.   Suboptimal positioning of the i-Gel® airway resulting in air entrainment.
e.   Use of low fresh gas flow.

1   Answer: A. The upper segment ends as a blind pouch and the lower segment communicates with the trachea.

The incidence of tracheo-oesophageal fistulae (TEF) is about 1 in 3000 to 4000 live births. It results from failure of the oesophagus and trachea to completely separate during development. There are several anatomical variations (Table 1). The most common type (85%) of lesion occurs when the lower segment communicates with the trachea and the upper end

Table 1. The anatomical characteristics of tracheo-oesophageal fistulae.

Anatomical type	%
Upper end blind pouch, lower end communicates with the trachea	85%
Both upper and lower segments end as blind pouches	8%
Two segments join together and communicate with the lower part of the trachea	4%
The upper segment communicates with the lower part of the trachea and the lower segment arises from the carina	1%
The upper segment communicates with the trachea and the lower segment ends as a blind pouch	1%

ends as a blind pouch. About 30% of babies are premature or have a low birth weight. There may be other associated congenital anomalies such as cardiac defects (ventricular septal defect, tetralogy of Fallot) and anorectal anomalies. The diagnosis is suspected by a history of maternal polyhydramnios.

The TEF can be confirmed by the inability to pass a suction catheter to the stomach or by the presence of air in the stomach on a chest X-ray taken soon after birth.

Further reading

1. Sharma S, Duerksen D. Tracheoesophageal fistula. http://emedicine.medscape.com/article/186735-overview.

2   Answer: E. Catheter infection.

Venous catheter infection is the most common complication associated with total parenteral nutrition (TPN) and bacteraemia/sepsis is the most serious complication of intravenous feeding. There is an increased incidence of pneumonia and sepsis in patients receiving TPN. Clinically significant liver disease may develop in about 5% of adults following long-term TPN. Liver disease progressing to cirrhosis and portal hypertension is more common in children. Abnormal liver function such as increases in alkaline phosphatase, transaminase, and raised bilirubin may also be seen. Osteoporosis and osteomalacia are additional complications associated with long-term TPN. The other metabolic complications include hyperglycaemia, hypoglycaemia, hyperkalaemia, hypokalaemia, hypophosphataemia and metabolic acidosis.

Further reading

1. Forbes A. Parenteral nutrition. *Current Opinion Gastroenterology* 2007; 23: 183-6.
2. Pittiruti M, Hamilton H, Biffi R, *et al.* ESPEN Guidelines on Parenteral Nutrition: Central Venous Catheter (access, care, diagnosis and therapy of complications). *Clinical Nutrition* 2009; 28: 365-77.
3. Hinds C, Watson D, Eds. Nutritional support. In: A *concise text book of intensive care.* Saunders Elsevier, 3rd ed, 2008; Chapter 11: 301-9.

3   Answer: C. Withdraw the needle and redirect more medially.

During a spinal anaesthetic procedure, if the needle deviates laterally and hits the nerve root, patients can experience sharp stabbing pain in the leg on the same side. The best option is to withdraw the needle and redirect it more medially away from the affected side to ensure that the needle is in the midline. Patients may also feel pain when the needle passes through the muscle on either side of the ligaments. Again, redirecting the needle away from the side of the pain or injecting local anaesthetic can be helpful.

Further reading
1. Casey WF. Spinal anaesthesia - a practical guide. Anaesthesia update, 2000, issue 12, article e8. http://www.nda.ox.ac.uk/wfsa /html/u12/u1208_05.htm.

4   Answer: B. Increased sympathetic discharge to peripheral vessels.

Blood flow to skeletal muscle rises significantly (up to 30-fold) in a rhythmically contracting muscle. Blood flow can increase at or even before the start of exercise. The initial rise is probably mediated via a neural response. Impulses in a sympathetic vasodilator system may be involved. Blood flow in resting muscles doubles after sympathectomy. Once exercise starts, local mechanisms maintain the high blood flow. There is no difference in flow in normal and sympathectomised individuals during exercise.

Further reading
1. Ganong WF, Ed. Sympathetic vasodilator system. In: *Review of medical physiology*, 22nd ed. New York, USA: McGraw Hill, 2005; Chapter 31: 609-10.

5   Answer: B. Systemic veins.

Normally, at rest, 50% of the circulating blood volume is in the systemic veins. Veins are partially collapsed and a large volume of fluid can be added to the circulation before the veins become distended to the point where further increments in volume produces a significant rise in venous pressure. For this reason the veins are called capacitance vessels.

Further reading

1. Ganong WF, Ed. Resistance and capacitance vessels. In: *Review of medical physiology*, 22nd ed. New York, USA: McGraw Hill, 2005; Chapter 30: 586-7.

6   Answer: B. Rocuronium 0.9mg/kg.

Suxamethonium is the most commonly used muscle relaxant for rapid sequence induction due to its rapid onset which achieves good intubating conditions. Rocuronium can be used as an alternative to suxamethonium. The blood results are suggestive of an atypical homozygous cholinesterase enzyme. If suxamethonium is administered it will cause prolonged apnoea lasting for several hours. Rocuronium has a rapid onset of action, which is dependent on the dose. A dose of 0.9mg/kg provides optimum intubating conditions at 45 seconds. Rocuronium does not have any cardiovascular side effects and a satisfactory reversal can be achieved with neostigmine. A rapid reversal can also be achieved using sugammadex.

Table 2. Onset of action of rocuronium.

Dose	Time to intubation
0.3mg/kg	120-150 seconds
0.45mg/kg	90 seconds
0.6mg/kg	60 seconds
0.9mg/kg	45 seconds

A systematic review concluded that suxamethonium produces superior intubation conditions to rocuronium when comparing both excellent and clinically acceptable intubating conditions.

Further reading

1. Perry JJ, Lee JS, Sillberg VA, Wells GA. Rocuronium versus succinylcholine for rapid sequence induction intubation. *Cochrane Database Syst Rev* 2008; CD002788.

7 Answer: D. Fentanyl.

Chest wall rigidity has been associated with potent opioids such as fentanyl and remifentanil. Although it is associated with rapid intravenous administration of a high dose of fentanyl, it has been also reported following aliquots of 50μg of fentanyl. Muscle rigidity observed with fentanyl has been antagonised by levallorphan. Thiopental sodium has been used to blunt the degree of muscle rigidity associated with high-dose fentanyl. A severe degree of muscle rigidity at induction may require a rapidly-acting muscle relaxant such as suxamethonium.

Priming with vecuronium (0.02mg/kg) or rocuronium (0.06mg/kg) has been shown to reduce muscle rigidity associated with remifentanil. Midazolam at a dose of 0.075mg/kg has been shown to attenuate chest wall muscle rigidity, but it does not prevent it.

Further reading

1. Vaughn RL, Bennett CR. Fentanyl chest wall rigidity syndrome - a case report. *Anesthesia Progress* 1981; 28: 50-1.
2. Vacant CA, Silbert BS, Vacanti FX. The effects of thiopental sodium on fentanyl-induced muscle rigidity in a human model. *Journal of Clinical Anaesthesia* 1991; 3: 395-8.
3. Nakada J, Nishira M, Hosoda R, *et al.* Priming with rocuronium or vecuronium prevents remifentanil-mediated muscle rigidity and difficult ventilation. *Journal of Clinical Anaesthesia* 2009; 23: 323-8.

8   Answer: E. Halothane.

Mean arterial pressure (MAP) decreases with increasing concentration of desflurane, sevoflurane, isoflurane, halothane, and enflurane in a dose-dependent manner. With the exception of halothane, the decrease in the MAP primarily reflects a decrease in systemic vascular resistance (SVR) versus a decrease in cardiac output. In contrast, halothane decreases MAP almost entirely by a decrease in cardiac output with little change in SVR. A dose-related fall in SVR by inhalational agents is minimised by the substitution of nitrous oxide for a portion of inhalational agent.

Further reading

1. Reichle FM, Conzen PF. Halogenated inhalational anaesthetics. *Best Pract Res Clin Anaesthesiol* 2003; 17(1): 29-46.

9   Answer: B. Bupivacaine > lignocaine > prilocaine > procaine.

The duration of action of local anaesthetic is related to its structure, primarily to the length of the intermediate chain joining the aromatic and amine groups. However, it should be noted that protein binding is an important determinant of duration of action of the drug. Clearly the molecular structure of the drug affects its protein-binding ability. Therefore, all local anaesthetics differ in the extent to which they are protein-bound. So, for example, lignocaine is approximately 65% protein bound, whereas bupivacaine is 95% protein bound. Therefore, bupivacaine will have a longer duration of action than lignocaine - which is in fact the case. Procaine (an ester), in contrast, is only 6% protein bound and has a very short duration of action. Differences in protein binding also result in differing duration of unwanted side effects and are one of the reasons that bupivacaine is considered more toxic than lignocaine.

Further reading

1. Heavner JE. Local anesthetics. *Curr Opin Anaesthesiol* 2007; 20(4): 336-42.

10 Answer: A. It increases methaemoglobinaemia.

The treatment of cyanide poisoning includes supportive care: airway control, ventilation, 100% oxygen delivery, crystalloids and vasopressors as needed for hypotension. Activated charcoal should be given after oral exposure in alert patients who are able to protect their airway or after endotracheal intubation in unconscious patients. Hydroxocobalamin should be administered if the diagnosis is strongly suspected, without waiting for laboratory confirmation. Hydroxocobalamin combines with cyanide to form cyanocobalamin (vitamin B12), which is renally excreted. Co-administration of sodium thiosulfate has been suggested to have a synergic effect on detoxification. Sodium nitrite induces methaemoglobin in red blood cells, which combines with cyanide, thus releasing cytochrome oxidase enzyme. Sodium thiosulfate enhances the conversion of cyanide to thiocyanate, which is renally excreted. Thiosulfate has a delayed effect and is typically used with sodium nitrite for faster antidote action.

Further reading
1. Bebarta VS, Tanen DA, *et al.* Hydroxocobalamin and sodium thiosulfate versus sodium nitrite and sodium thiosulfate in the treatment of acute cyanide toxicity in a swine model. *Annals of Emergency Medicine* 2010; 55: 345-51.

11 Answer: C. Performing a three-point calibration.

In order to obtain an accurate blood pressure reading, the system should be appropriately calibrated. Zero calibration eliminates the effect of atmospheric pressure on the measured pressure. Zeroing ensures that the monitor indicates zero pressure in the absence of applied pressure; it eliminates the offset drift (zero drift). To eliminate the gradient drift, calibration at a higher pressure is necessary. For applying a known higher pressure, the transducer is connected to an aneroid manometer using sterile tubing through a three-way stopcock and the manometer pressure is raised to 100 and 200mm Hg. The monitor display should read the same pressure as that applied to the transducer.

For accurate measurement the transducer system must be 'zeroed' to a reference point. This reference point is usually on the left side in the mid-axillary line at the level of the left ventricle.

Referencing or levelling the transducer system is accomplished by aligning the air-fluid interface of the transducer system (the three-way stopcock at the top of the transducer) to the mid-axillary point. Zeroing is then performed by opening the three-way stopcock between the patient and the transducer to atmosphere and selecting the zero on the monitor.

In the supine position, the mid-axillary line is an appropriate reference point. Raising or lowering the transducer above or below this point will result in an error equivalent to 7.5mm Hg for each 10cm change in the height. However, if the clinician is interested in measuring the MAP at the level of the brain in the sitting position, then a different reference point should be chosen.

Generation of a square wave at the catheter tip is the gold standard laboratory test in assessing the dynamic response of a monitoring system. It is used for assessing the optimum damping coefficient.

Further reading
1. Davis PD, Kenny GNC. Presentation and handling of data and basic measurement concepts. *Basic physics and measurement in anaesthesia*, 5th ed. London, UK: Butterworth-Heinemann, 2003; Chapter 25: 285-8.
2. Kleinman B, Powell S, Gardner RM. Equivalence of fast flush and square wave testing of blood pressure monitoring systems. *Journal of Clinical Monitoring* 1996; 12: 149-54.

12 Answer: B. Mapleson A system.

According to the modified Mapleson classification, there are six different types of breathing systems (Mapleson A through F). They can be arranged in the order of A, B, C, D, E and F, according to the requirement of fresh gas flow (FGF) to prevent rebreathing during spontaneous ventilation; Mapleson A requires the minimum and Mapleson F requires the maximum FGF. They all contain similar components, which include a fresh gas flow inlet, corrugated tubing, reservoir bag and unidirectional valve. They are assembled in different sequences.

In a Mapleson A system, the expiratory valve is located near the patient end and the fresh gas flow inlet is located proximal to the reservoir bag. This arrangement is most efficient for CO_2 elimination during spontaneous ventilation. As inhalational induction requires spontaneous ventilation and a high concentration of volatile anaesthetic, it is more economical to use a Mapleson A breathing system as compared to the other systems. During controlled ventilation, the expiratory valve is closed to permit manual ventilation of the lungs. This system is less efficient during controlled ventilation.

In a Mapleson D system, the position of the expiratory valve and fresh gas flow inlet are reversed, enabling it to be the most efficient system for controlled ventilation.

Further reading
1. Davey AJ. Breathing system and their components. In: *Ward's anaesthetic equipment*, 5th ed, Davey AJ, Diba A, Eds. Philadelphia, USA: Elsevier Saunders, 2005; Chapter 8: 3.

13 Answer: C. Minimum alveolar concentration (MAC) of volatile anaesthetic agent.

The isolated forearm technique is a crude method of monitoring the depth of anaesthesia. It is not used in current clinical practice. Before the administration of muscle relaxants, a tourniquet applied to the patient's upper arm is inflated above systolic blood pressure. Movement of the arm either spontaneously or to command indicates wakefulness. Its clinical use is limited by the duration of the tourniquet, as prolonged application of tourniquets can result in ischaemia of the arm.

There is limited clinical evidence to support that using the bispectral index reduces the incidence of awareness. It allows close titration of both volatile and intravenous anaesthetic agents. This may ensure a faster emergence and lower cost. Potentially, this may increase the risk of awareness.

Once equilibrium is achieved between the alveoli, blood and brain, the minimum alveolar concentration (MAC) is the best available method to monitor continuous brain concentration of volatile anaesthetics. The MAC awake is the minimum alveolar concentration of volatile anaesthetic required for producing unconsciousness in 50% of subjects.

Lower oesophageal contractility is measured using a balloon in the lower oesophagus. The amplitude and latency of both spontaneous and provoked oesophageal contractions is reduced under general anaesthesia.

Late cortical responses originate from the frontal cortex and are abolished by sedatives, hence, they are not useful in monitoring depth of anaesthesia.

Further reading

1. Sice PJA. Depth of anaesthesia. Anaesthesia update, 2005; 19: article 10. http://www.nda.ox.ac.uk/wfsa/html/u19/u1910_01.htm.

14   Answer: C. Platinum resistance thermometer.

A resistance thermometer displays a linear increase in resistance with increasing temperature. Over the range of 0-100°C, the change in resistance is linearly related to the change in temperature. The platinum wire resistance thermometer can measure a very small change in temperature up to +/-0.0001°C. The main disadvantage is slow response time.

The infrared thermometer absorbs infrared radiation emitted by the body and converts the infrared signal into an electrical signal.

The mercury thermometer is not as accurate as the electronic methods.

Thermistors are made of semiconductor beads and contain a Wheatstone bridge circuit. The resistance of the thermistor decreases non-linearly with increasing temperature. They accurately measure the temperature to an order of 0.1°C.

The Bourdon gauge thermometer is relatively simple, robust and cheap, but not very accurate.

Further reading

1. Stoker RM. Measuring temperature. *Anaesthesia and Intensive Care Medicine* 2005; 6: 194-8.

15   Answer: B. Facial nerve and orbicularis occuli.

Orbicularis oculi has a good blood supply. Therefore, the onset and offset of the block is faster in this muscle compared to peripheral muscles. The laryngeal muscles behave as central muscles for onset of the block. The onset of block is best monitored by stimulation of the facial nerve.

The peripheral nerve chosen for monitoring neuromuscular block (NMB) should be superficial with a motor component which needs to be easily accessible.

Further reading
1. Hunter JM, McGrath CD. Monitoring of neuromuscular block. *British Journal of Anaesthesia CEACCP* 2006; 6: 7-12.
2. Sardesai AM, Griffiths R. Monitoring techniques: neuromuscular blockade. *Anaesthesia and Intensive Care Medicine* 2005; 6: 198-9.
3. Hemmerling TM, Donati F. Neuromuscular blockade at the larynx, the diaphragm and the corrugator supercilii muscle: a review. *Canadian Journal of Anaesthesia* 2003; 50: 779-94.

16   Answer: C. Medium-sized bronchi.

Between the trachea and the alveolar sacs, the airways divide 23 times. The first 16 generations of the passages form the conducting zone, which transports gas from and to the exterior. They are made up of bronchi, bronchioles, and terminal bronchioles. The remaining seven generations form the transitional and respiratory zones where gas exchange occurs. They are made up of respiratory bronchioles, alveolar ducts, and alveoli. Multiple divisions greatly increase the total cross-sectional area of the airways, from $2.5cm^2$ in the trachea to $11,800cm^2$ in the alveoli. Based on Poiseuille's equation, it is obvious that the resistance is greatest in the very narrow airways, but direct measurement has revealed a greater proportion of the resistance contributed by the medium-sized bronchi.

Further reading
1. Ganong WF, Ed. Anatomy of lungs. In: *Review of medical physiology*, 22nd ed. New York, USA: McGraw Hill, 2005; Chapter 34: 649-50.

17 Answer: B. The pH of his blood is likely to fall more slowly than the pH of his CSF.

The blood brain barrier is readily permeable to CO_2. Any rise in blood CO_2 readily penetrates the blood brain barrier and enters the CSF. CO_2 that enters the CSF is readily rehydrated. The H_2CO_3 dissociates and local H^+ concentration rises. The H^+ concentration in the brain interstitial fluid parallels arterial PCO_2. Secondly, the buffer system in the CSF is not as efficient as that in the blood. Therefore, pH changes are more marked in CSF with a respiratory acidosis.

Further reading

1. Ganong WF, Ed. Chemical control of breathing. In: *Review of medical physiology*, 22nd ed. New York, USA: McGraw-Hill, 2005; Chapter 36: 672-8.

18 Answer: A. Increased urinary ammonium excretion.

Renal acid secretion is affected by changes in the intracellular PCO_2, K^+ concentration, carbonic anhydrase level and adrenocortical hormone concentration. In respiratory acidosis, more intracellular H_2CO_3 is available to buffer the hydroxyl ions and acid secretion increases. In metabolic acidosis, ammonium (NH_4^+) excretion increases. Normally, NH_4^+ is in equilibrium with ammonia (NH_3) and H^+ in the renal tubular cells. The pKa of this reaction is 9.0. Therefore, the ratio of NH_3 to NH_4^+ at a pH of 7.0 is 1:100. But NH_3 is lipid-soluble and diffuses across cell membranes down its concentration gradient into the interstitial fluid and tubular urine. In urine, it reacts with H^+ to form NH_4^+. This NH_4^+ remains in the urine.

Further reading

1. Ganong WF, Ed. Acidification of the urine and bicarbonate excretion. In: *Review of medical physiology*, 22nd ed. New York, USA: McGraw-Hill, 2005; Chapter 38: 720-2.

19 Answer: A. Thalassaemia.

There are two major types of inherited disorders of haemoglobin in humans. Haemoglobinopathies, in which abnormal polypeptide chains are produced, and thalassaemias, in which the chains are normal in structure, but are produced in reduced amounts or are absent because of defects in the regulatory portion of the globin genes.

Further reading
1. Ganong WF, Ed. Haemoglobin. In: *Review of medical physiology*, 22nd ed. New York, USA: McGraw-Hill, 2005; Chapter 27: 534-7.

20 Answer: E. Hypothyroidism due to a primary abnormality in the hypothalamus.

The symptoms and signs of this woman suggest that she is suffering from hypothyroidism. TSH levels rising after administration of TRH indicates that endogenous TRH production is deficient. TRH is produced by the hypothalamus. Therefore, this patient has a primary abnormality in the hypothalamus. TSH is produced by the anterior pituitary.

Further reading
1. Ganong WF, Ed. Regulation of thyroid secretion. In: *Review of medical physiology*, 22nd ed. New York, USA: McGraw-Hill, 2005; Chapter 18: 326-8.

21 Answer: A. Hyponatraemia.

Diuretic drugs are one of the common causes of hyponatraemia. This patient is on a combination of two diuretics.

Bendrofluazide is a thiazide diuretic. Thiazides reduce the sodium re-absorption at the cortical diluting segment of the distal tubule. They also stimulate potassium secretion at the distal tubule.

Amiloride is a potassium-sparing diuretic. It acts on the collecting tubule by increasing sodium loss and reducing potassium loss. It does not antagonise the action of aldosterone. Therefore, it is complementary to thiazide diuretics.

Both drugs cause urinary sodium loss. In addition, the potassium-sparing effect of amiloride aggravates thiazide-induced hyponatraemia by retaining potassium and exchanging sodium for hydrogen ions. Most cases of thiazide-induced hyponatremia occur in elderly patients, with a female predominance.

Thiazide diuretics are water-soluble and are rapidly excreted by active secretion in the proximal tubule. Thiazides and uric acid are secreted through the same mechanism in the renal tubules. This competition leads to a reduction in uric acid secretion and, thus, elevated plasma levels of uric acid. Other biochemical abnormalities observed with the use of these diuretics are: hypokalaemia, hypomagnesaemia and alkalosis. Thiazides cause hypercalcaemia whilst loop diuretics may cause hypocalcaemia.

Further reading
1. Peck TE, Hill SA, Williams M, Eds. Diuretics. In: *Pharmacology for anaesthesia and intensive care*, 3rd ed. Cambridge, UK: Cambridge University Press, 2008; Chapter 21: 305-10.
2. Liamis G, Miloonis H, Elisaf M. A review of drug-induced hyponatraemia. *American Journal of Kidney Diseases* 2008; 52: 144-53.

22 Answer: A. Prednisolone 15mg on the morning of surgery.

Those patients taking more than 10mg of prednisolone a day need their routine pre-operative dose of steroid or hydrocortisone 25mg IV at induction for minor surgery. This patient is having minor surgery; routine pre-operative steroid cover is sufficient.

During prolonged therapy with corticosteroids, adrenal atrophy develops. Abrupt withdrawal can lead to acute adrenal insufficiency. To compensate for diminished adrenocortical response caused by prolonged corticosteroid treatment, significant intercurrent illness, trauma or surgical procedures, there should be a temporary increase in the dose. Any patient taking more than 10mg of prednisolone a day would require supplementary hydrocortisone during the peri-operative period.

For minor surgery, the usual oral corticosteroid dose on the morning of the surgery or hydrocortisone 25-50mg intravenously at induction is sufficient. The usual oral corticosteroid dose is recommenced after surgery.

For moderate or major surgery, the usual oral corticosteroid dose is given on the morning of surgery and hydrocortisone 25mg intravenously at induction, followed by hydrocortisone 25mg three times a day by intravenous injection for 24 hours after moderate surgery or for 48-72 hours after major surgery. The usual pre-operative oral corticosteroid dose is recommenced on stopping hydrocortisone injections.

Further reading

1. Joint Formulary Committee. *British National Formulary*, 58th ed. London, UK: British Medical Association and Royal Pharmaceutical Society of Great Britain, 2009.
2. Davies M, Hardman J. Anaesthesia and adrenocortical disease. *British Journal of Anaesthesia CEACCP* 2005; 5: 122-6.
3. Nicholson G, Burrin JM, Hall GM. Peri-operative steroid supplementation. *Anaesthesia* 1998; 53: 1091-104.
4. Blanshard H. Patient on steroids - endocrine and metabolic disease. In: *Oxford handbook of anaesthesia*. Oxford, UK: Oxford University Press, 2006; Chapter 8: 166-7.

23 Answer: E. Atracurium.

Both vecuronium and rocuronium are steroidal muscle relaxants. They undergo hepatic metabolism and elimination, hence, their clearance and elimination half-life is prolonged in liver disease resulting in prolonged neuromuscular blockade.

The elimination half-life of pancuronium is increased in cirrhosis due to the associated increase in the volume of distribution.

Plasma cholinesterase activity is reduced in patients with liver disease, prolonging the duration of mivacurium.

Atracurium undergoes organ independent Hofmann elimination (non-specific ester hydrolysis); therefore, its half-life and duration of action are not affected.

Although laudanosine, a metabolite of both atracurium and cis-atracurium, is eliminated primarily by the liver, the level is clinically insignificant to cause any neurotoxicity.

Further reading
1. Rothenberg DM, O'Connor CJ, Tuman KJ. Anesthesia and the hepatobiliary system. In: *Miller's anesthesia*, Volume 2, 7th ed. Miller RD, Ed. Philadelphia, USA: Churchill Livingstone, 2010; Chapter 66: 2139-40.
2. Vaja R, McNicol R, Sisley I. Anaesthesia for patients with liver disease. *British Journal of Anaesthesia CEACCP* 2010; 10: 15-9.

24 Answer: A. Intravenous 10ml of 10% calcium chloride over 5 minutes.

This patient has a high potassium level secondary to renal failure and ECG manifestations of hyperkalaemia. If this is not treated immediately it can result in life-threatening arrhythmias which include ventricular fibrillation. Calcium chloride protects the myocardium against arrhythmias due to high levels of potassium. 50ml of 50% glucose should be administered with insulin 10 units to reduce the levels of plasma potassium. Both insulin and salbutamol facilitate movement of potassium into the cell. Furosemide causes diuresis with potassium loss. Most importantly this patient requires haemodialysis to correct the hyperkalaemia.

Further reading
1. Singer M, Webb A. Metabolic disorders. In: *Oxford handbook of critical care*. New York, USA: Oxford University Press, 2008: 420-1.

25 Answer: C. Intravenous sugammadex 16mg/kg.

Sugammadex is used for the reversal of neuromuscular blockade caused by rocuronium and vecuronium. For reversal of routine neuromuscular block, sugammadex 2-4mg/kg may be used, but for the immediate reversal of neuromuscular blockade, a dose of 16mg/kg is required. Neostigmine and glycopyrrolate can be used for routine reversal of neuromuscular block, but not for reversal of profound neuromuscular block. The correct dose of neostigmine is 0.05-0.07mg/kg and of glycopyrrolate 0.01mg/kg. Edrophonium is not suitable for the given situation and is not usually used for reversal in clinical anaesthetic practice. It is used to differentiate a myasthenia crisis from a cholinergic crisis.

Further reading
1. Chambers D, Poulden M, *et al.* Sugammadex for reversal of neuromuscular block after rapid sequence intubation: a systematic review and economic assessment. *British Journal of Anaesthesia* 2010; 105(5): 568-75.
2. Wilkes AR. Heat and moisture exchangers and breathing system filters: their use in anaesthesia and intensive care Part 2 - practical use, including problems, and their use with paediatric patients. *Anaesthesia* 2011; 66: 40-51.

26 Answer: D. 4%.

As the atmospheric pressure is reduced, the delivered concentration is increased from that marked on the dial of a vaporiser. Since the barometric pressure is reduced by half of that at sea level, the concentration of vapour output doubles. However, anaesthetic action depends on the alveolar partial pressure, and not on concentration. The partial pressure of isoflurane delivered would be approximately the same at both altitudes since 2% isoflurane at 760mm Hg (15.2mm Hg) is the same as 4% isoflurane at 380mm Hg (15.2mm Hg). Saturated vapour pressure (SVP) is unaffected by atmospheric pressure and therefore the partial pressure of isoflurane delivered is the same as at sea level.

Further reading
1. Carter JA. Provision of anaesthesia in difficult situations and the developing world. In: *Ward's anaesthetic equipment*, 5th ed. Davey AJ, Diba A, Eds. Philadelphia, USA: Elsevier Saunders, 2005; Chapter 29: 485-98.

27 Answer: D. 400J.

A defibrillator is an instrument in which electric charge is stored and then released in a controlled fashion. The key component for storing the charge is a capacitor. The stored energy can be calculated using the following formula:

Stored energy, $E = \frac{1}{2} QV$ where Q is the charge and V is the voltage.

In this example, Energy $= \frac{1}{2} \times 0.2 \times 4000V = 400J$

The maximum delivered energy is 360J. Defibrillators also have a lower minimum setting, normally 100J, for use with internal cardiac electrodes in a patient with an open chest.

Further reading
1. Davis PD, Kenny GNC. Electricity. In: *Basic physics and measurement in anaesthesia*, 5th ed. London, UK; Butterworth Heinemann, 2003; Chapter 14: 157-8.

28 Answer: D. Improved airway seal, enabling positive pressure ventilation.

A Proseal® LMA (PLMA), like the classic LMA, consists of an airway tube, bowl and cuff. The airway tube is shorter but is reinforced to a similar calibre of an equivalent flexible LMA.

The modifications compared to the classic LMA are:

◆ Larger and deeper bowl with no grille.
◆ Posterior extension of the mask cuff.
◆ Oesophageal drain tube running parallel to the airway tube and exiting at the mask tip.
◆ Integral silicone bite block.
◆ Anterior pocket for seating an introducer or finger during insertion.

When the PLMA is correctly positioned, the cuff tip lies behind the cricoid cartilage at the origin of the oesophagus. In the event of regurgitation, the liquid and semi-solid contents may be aspirated through the drain port. The haemodynamic response to insertion or removal of a PLMA is the same as that for a classic LMA. The posterior cuff and the increased bulk of the PLMA mask together substantially increase the pharyngeal leak pressure and reduce the risk of gastric insufflation during positive pressure ventilation. The airway tube of the PLMA is shorter than the classic LMA, but is wire-reinforced and of similar calibre to the flexible LMA. Airway resistance is 20% greater than the classic LMA. The patient in the above mentioned scenario would need to be in the lithotomy position with anaesthetic duration of more than an hour and, hence, controlled ventilation is preferable. The aspiration risk is not high as this is an elective procedure in a fit and well patient. An airway device which can facilitate controlled ventilation with minimal leak and risk of gastric insufflation, such as a PLMA, would be the right choice for this procedure.

Further reading
1. Cook T, Howes B. Supraglottic airway devices: recent advances. *British Journal of Anaesthesia CEACCP* 2011; 11: 56-61.

29 Answer: A. Peripheral oxygen saturation.

The extent of sensory block can be assessed by checking touch and pain sensation. ECG monitoring can detect a block involving the thoracic sympathetic fibres, which will result in bradycardia. Peripheral oxygen saturation will only decrease at a late stage, in high block, due to hypoventilation. Respiratory depression associated with significant sedation can also result in hypoxia.

BIS monitoring will assess the level of sedation, which is again related to the height of sensory block. The mechanism involved in producing sedation during spinal anaesthesia includes the systemic effects of absorbed local anaesthetics and the rostral spread of local anaesthetic through the cerebrospinal fluid with direct action on the brain.

Further reading
1. Iida R, Iwasaki K, Kato J, Ogawa S. Bispectral index is related to the spread of spinal sensory block in patients with combined general and spinal anaesthesia. *British Journal of Anaesthesia* 2011; 106: 202-7.

30 Answer: D. Suboptimal positioning of the i-Gel® airway resulting in air entrainment.

Suboptimal insertion of an i-Gel® airway results in the gastric channel being open to the larynx. In a spontaneously breathing patient, air can be entrained through the gastric channel which dilutes the anaesthetic gases. As this happens downstream to the point of agent monitoring (near the catheter mount), the inspired concentration reading is not affected.

The patient has been anaesthetised for approximately one hour; equilibration between the alveolar and brain concentrations of sevoflurane should have occurred. Therefore, there should be no gross difference between inspired and expired concentrations despite low fresh gas flow.

Malfunctioning of the vaporiser would result in inaccurate vapour delivery. In this scenario the inspired concentration closely resembles the dial setting. The use of low fresh gas flow is likely to result in a gross difference between the dial setting and inspired concentration measured by the agent analyser.

Further reading
1. Intersurgical Ltd. Intersurgical i-Gel® User Guide, Issue 5. Wokingham, UK: Intersurgical Ltd, 2008.
2. Baxter S. Phenomenon with i-gel airway? *Anaesthesia* 2008; 63: 1265.